A YAK IN THE FRIDGE

Life and Work in Nepal

John Dickinson and Family

Aided and abetted by
Angela Dickinson
James Dickinson
Mary Probyn

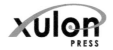

Contents

Dedication

To the People of Nepal

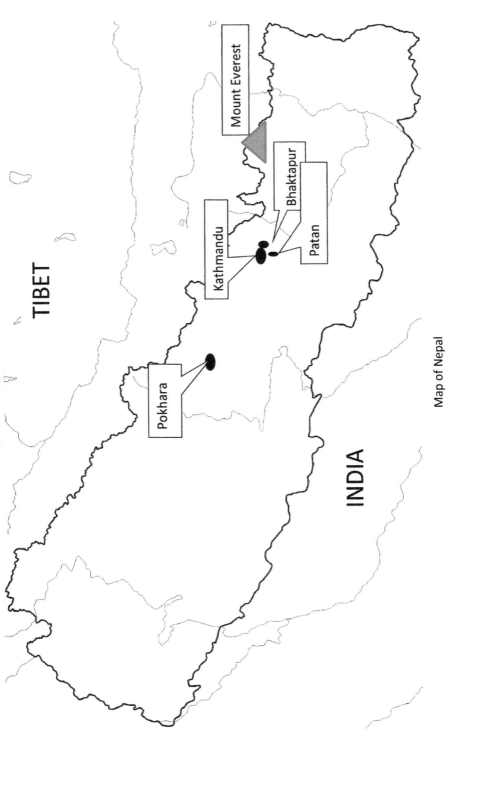

Map of Nepal

Introduction

I offer this book, written with a lot of help from my family, reflecting on the best part of a lifetime working as a doctor in the Himalayan Kingdom of Nepal. It is not an autobiography of the "I was born at a very early age..." sort, but more a series of anecdotes that might or might not be called memoirs. They centre not on me, but on the land and people of Nepal.

It is not a complete political, geographical or historical study of Nepal, but there are elements of this. I have made an attempt to portray society and the practice of medicine as it was for me in the Nepal of 40-odd years ago and the way it has changed. It will also show how the whole nation has developed, and contrast the quaint old-fashioned-ness of the 1960s and 70s with the modern state. (For example, it is not a Kingdom anymore!) I hope to give the reader an impression of some of the fascinating and colourful people, Nepalese and others, who have crossed my path over the years.

It will not take you long to realise that we went and worked with a Christian mission, but this is not a 'missionary book'. There is no attempt to explain or justify mission, to give a history of mission in Nepal, (Lindell, 1979) or even to chronicle in detail the extraordinary growth of the Nepali Church. Both have been done competently elsewhere. These things form a background to the theme and should be accepted for what they are. Some stories will reveal my own personal faith and my identification with the mission statement of the United Mission to Nepal under which we worked; "To serve the people of Nepal in the name and spirit of Jesus Christ and to make him known by word and life." There is some consideration of the different world views represented by Hinduism and Christianity, with some analysis of the ways they differ and misunderstand one another, but I hope that Hindus, Buddhists, Christians and those with other faiths or none will feel comfortable reading this book.

Needless to say, we have different memories and different perceptions, so I have encouraged the rest of the family, not only to write chapters, but to make different sorts of interjections in the text of all and any of the other chapters. These appear in square brackets.

Who were we in 1969 when we went to Nepal? And who are we now in 2015?

John was the father, a young doctor with a recent MRCP qualification and a new Diploma in Theology. *Now* he is grizzled, retired from clinical medicine but teaching part time in the Leeds and, until recently, Hull York Medical Schools, sometimes visiting Nepal to teach in medical schools there. For years he has been known as 'Hop' to the rest of the family.

Angela was the mother, a graduate teacher of French with experience of an innovative programme of teaching French in primary schools. However, she was determined to make family her first priority. *Now* she is retired, a teacher of English as a second language, sometimes with Gurkha families in Catterick, sometimes in a Nursing School in Nepal. She answers to 'Nana' and still makes family her first priority!

Mary Joy was a three year old. *Now* she is a general practitioner in Hertfordshire, wife of Andy and mother of Isabel and Abby. She dropped the 'Joy' along the way, at least partly because people kept getting it wrong. She is author of a novel based on the Kumari culture of the Newars in Kathmandu, 'The Living Goddess'. (Probyn, 2011)

Jamie was a one year old in a carrycot. Now, he is an Advisory Teacher in Speech and Language to Hertfordshire Education Authority, married to Caroline and father of Max. He has always been the joker of the family and tops his father by at least two inches at 6'3".

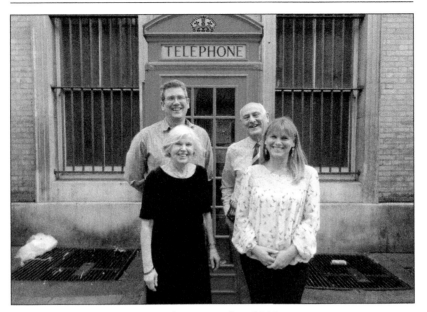

London December 2015

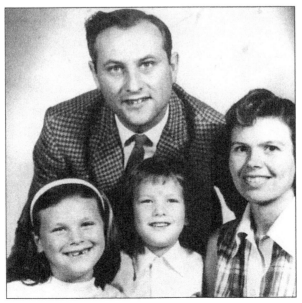

Family circa 1973

Chapter 1.

Going to Nepal

The day before departure from England in September 1969, 3 year old Mary Joy was being fitted for some new shoes. "I'm going to Kathmandu tomorrow" she said brightly to the saleslady.

"Yes, dear, and I'm going to Timbuktu." came the answer!

But we were! We were about to join United Mission to Nepal sent by the Bible and Medical Missionary Fellowship to serve in the Shanta Bhawan Hospital. UMN over the years has had up to 40 contributing missions in 20 different countries.

Two days later found us alighting from the plane in the Kathmandu Valley. The airport, now known as the Tribhuwan International Airport, was then often called "*Gaucher*", for that was what it had been, a cow field. Even at that time, cows would sometimes have to be shooed off the runway. This runway was generally too short for jets, but Thai Airways began operating a Caravelle from Bangkok,which could only land by throwing out a parachute to help it slow to taxiing speed. Planes were always entertaining, but the parachute plane was the big attraction for the public on a Sunday afternoon.

Imagine the family of four, descending the ramp into that primitive air field. I had a basic medical qualification under my belt and also a higher one (MRCP for those who know these things). I probably felt ready for anything, but time will tell that I wasn't! Angela had degrees from Oxford like me and a Diploma of Education. She had experience of an innovative scheme teaching French to Primary

School children in Banbury, but at this time was focussed on being a mother to the children, which proved just as well. Mary Joy was the three year old and Jamie was the baby in the carry cot. For people like us, carry cots were a good way of carrying supplies surplus to the luggage allowance, but we knew one family who had the carry cot so stuffed with possessions that the baby actually fell out!

We were met by friends, which is always re-assuring, particularly as we had had a tiring and tricky journey via Cairo, Bombay and New Delhi and had faced for the first time the chaos of coolies, taxi drivers and crowds that is Delhi. Our drive to the UMN mission guest house took us on narrow, pot-holed roads, puddled by the monsoon rains, and past the characteristic pagoda-shaped temples of Nepal. I could smell wood smoke, pungently bringing back my four months in West Africa. There were few private cars in those days and we had the extraordinary sight of taxis obligatorily painted with tiger stripes. The monsoon clouds were draped like shawls over the hills surrounding the Valley.

There are lots of memories of days in the guest house; learning to use mosquito nets, communal living, exotic plants in the garden, uncertain electricity and water shortage. (The rule for the W.C. was "If it's brown, flush it down. If it's yellow, let it mellow".)

We quickly learned of the change of the seasons in Nepal. The summer South East monsoon gave way dramatically within a few days of our arrival and the clouds over the mountains started to move in the opposite direction, from West to East. We newcomers climbed to the roof of the guest house at sunrise and sunset to catch our first glimpses of the Himalaya, the 'Home of Snow'. [*Note*: The plural 'Himalayas' is unnecessary.] Ganesh Himal, with its many summits and the dramatic Langtang Himal were among many that became old friends and landmarks to us. If the conditions were right, we could enjoy the 'alpenglow', the reds and oranges that that light up the snows as the sun rises and sets. There were just a few spots from which Everest was visible in the East.

The ensuing season was bright, warm and dry through October and the beginning of November. This is the season in which fall the great Hindu festivals of *Dashain* and *Tihar* (also known as *Diwali*). Soon, though, comes the winter of morning mists. Kathmandu is a bowl-like valley in which mists are trapped in a heavier, colder layer.

Meteorologists refer to this as an inversion phenomenon, I believe. As a result, the days start cold and misty and everyone is wrapped in shawls and sweaters, but the mist lifts mid-morning, the sun begins to warm the valley and sweaters are shed. In those days, there was very little heating available indoors, so people working in offices would take their papers to tables outside to keep warm. The advent of the ubiquitous computer sadly put a stop to this. [*Mary says:* Dad, Seriously?! It must have been most of 20 years after this that computers tipped up in Nepal!]

Towards the end of January come the Winter Rains, of which more later. Though cold and miserable, they are usually short–they last only a few days and may not come at all. Then there is a gradual warming, culminating in a hot and humid May and beginning of June and then the onset of the main monsoon season starting from about 16 June and lasting until the end of September. For those thinking of trekking, the ideal months are October–November and March–April, and these are also the mountaineering seasons, though the build-up of an expedition often has to start earlier.

I've used the western names for the months, but we had to get used to the Nepali Calendar, the *Bikram Sambat*. The 12 months are determined by the astrologers, so their lengths and equivalence to other calendars varies. Their names are *Baishakh, Jestha, Asar, Srawan, Bhadau, Asoj, Kartik, Mangsir, Poush, Magh, Falgun* and *Chaitra*. The first of *Baishakh* falls near the middle of our April and is the Nepali New Year's Day. (Incidentally, some Nepalese celebrate the Tibetan New Year and others the Newari New Year, so it's possible to have at least four New Year's Days.) To complicate it further, we went to Nepal at the end of September 1969 AD, which was near the middle of *Kartik* 2026 BS. Time travel as HG Wells didn't know it!

Language Study

We lived in the guest house for four months. [*Angela says:* We were looked after in the guest house by the wife of the director of UMN who was very helpful. When 35 years later I met two of their daughters, who had been at boarding school, she said: "I think you knew our parents better than we did".] This was for obligatory Nepali language study which took place sitting in the sun under poinsettias

17

with an excellent language teacher. Frustrating in the sense that I was eager to get to grips with treating patients, which is what I had come to do, but it was an essential prerequisite. It would be going too far to say that it is impossible to make a medical contribution without speaking the local language, because a number of our visitors did manage by using interpreters and sign language and advising less experienced doctors. But an on-going and meaningful relationship with patients is impossible without a common language, and English was an uncommon skill in Nepal in those days, being not even taught in government schools.

People have often asked me if Nepali was easy to learn. I usually reply that I'm still learning it! It is derived from Sanskrit and related to Hindi, Urdu and Bengali. The script is called Devanagri and some people, including British Gurkha Army officers, have tried to avoid it by using Romanised Nepali. I don't think this works except for very basic communication. One reason is that Devanagri is phonetic; in general, one symbol represents one sound and one sound only. Easier than English! If you know the symbol, you know how it should be pronounced. But it is essential to learn the letters of the alphabet and all the conjuncts; that is, the way they join together in a wealth of combinations.

Nepali consonants are written below a headline, with most vowels placed above or below the consonants. Verbs are placed at the ends of sentences and there are no definite or indefinite articles. 'Prepositions' are actually postpositions, coming at the ends of the nouns to which they refer. There are no definite or indefinite articles, though numbers may be used. So: "He one village to went".

Phonetic alphabet notwithstanding, pronunciation is perhaps the hardest aspect to master. When, on rare occasions, I can persuade the very polite and tolerant Nepalese to criticise my language skills, this is the area they focus on, even today. Aspiration–the addition of a puff of air to a consonant -makes a big difference to meaning. There are aspirated and un-aspirated forms of consonants equivalent to b, c, g, j, k and p. In addition, d and t have aspirated and un-aspirated forms and dental and palatal forms of each, so there are four 'd's and four 't's.

Then, it is important to remember that there are some 40 mother tongues in Nepal. Though most people speak Nepali as a *lingua franca*, they may speak a watered down form characteristic of their own caste or tribe. Because we were taught largely by Kathmandu Brahmins, Nepalese often say "You speak Nepali better than we do". This sounds very gratifying, but I think it means roughly that we speak more grammatically.

Recognising the importance of language, we tried to use it whenever possible. This often meant insisting on speaking Nepali with people whose English was perfectly good and haggling in the bazaar for things we had no intention of buying. Disgraceful! We also went to a Nepali church from the very first week we were there, even though there were services in English elsewhere. This meant understanding very little at first, but it helped with the language study and we intended to take a full part in church life.

By the time I started working in the hospital I could conduct consultations in Nepali and communicate with my Nepali colleagues. I still needed some help from interpreters from time to time and made some horrendous mistakes as you will see.

First Hospital Visits

I knew before we arrived that I would be assigned as Consultant Physician (at age 29!) to the Shanta Bhawan Hospital in Patan (across the Bagmati River from Kathmandu). However we were encouraged not to offer our services to our assigned post, but to concentrate on language study for the first four months. On the whole, I complied.

Dr Denis Roche had been running the UMN hospital at Bhaktapur, nine miles to the East, for some years. He handled everything that came along and made good progress in TB control. At weekends, I went to spend a day with him and apprentice myself to this very self-effacing but very effective senior man. He had some wonderful aphorisms, such as "Right lower lobe pneumonia in Nepal is amoebic liver abscess". Of course, it isn't, as he well knew, but it was great for remembering the possibility. Angela would likewise learn about housekeeping in Nepal from his wife Ann and the children would play with their four girls. There was a very experienced Swedish nurse at the hospital as well and a young Swedish nurse who was a fellow language student would sometimes come with us to spend time with

19

her. It was amusing to hear the Nepalis on the bus discussing whether she was my older or younger wife and who the children belonged to.

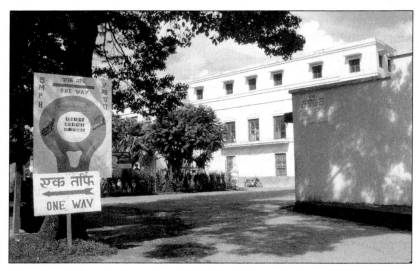

Shanta Bhawan Hospital. Photo: Dr Gerry Hankins

Denis had a very tiring job and, though he willingly acted as my mentor, sometimes he would simply go to bed and leave me to run the hospital, dealing with outpatients, emergencies and the wards. I felt totally inadequate, but I am glad to say there were no disasters.

As part of my orientation, I did visit my future hospital on a few occasions. Shanta Bhawan means "Palace of Peace", a good name for a hospital though in fact it got its name from General Shanta Shamsher Jung Bahadur Rana, son of a former ruler of Nepal in the period of Rana Prime Ministerships and puppet Shah kings. It had indeed been his palace, containing some 60 rooms. In 1956 it was converted for use as a hospital by some of the first Christian missionaries to enter the country after the overthrow of the Rana regime and restoration of power to the monarchy in the early 1950s. (Before that, there were virtually no foreigners allowed in the country.) In 1969, the Children's Ward, the Maternity Ward and the Nursing School were in Surendra Bhawan, a few hundred yards down the hill and named after another Rana General who was still living and became my patient. The wards moved to the main site a few years later following the building of *'Asha Niwas'*, the House of Hope. The Nursing School moved to yet another Rana palace, Nir Bhawan.

So I entered this majestic building with awe and great interest, noting its marble floors and wide staircases, becoming less imposing as one ascended to the former servants' quarters on the top floor. Needless to say, this was where my wards were!

One of the first things I did was a ward round with the two physicians, married to one another, whom I was to replace. Dr Peter and Dr Alice were German and I already had some idea that German medicine was rather different from what I was used to. This was confirmed when we saw several cases of viral meningitis, a small epidemic of a mild and self- healing condition. I noticed that they were all receiving antibiotics, though generally these are not effective in virus infections. Naturally I asked about this and was told "But you see zey always get better!"

I'm not sure how I could work with a medically qualified spouse in the same specialty. When we became engaged, Angela asked if I wanted her to re-train as a nurse. When I said that I didn't, she looked heartily relieved! But it seemed Dr Peter and Dr Alice got on very well, though the nurses found it confusing when they would go round the patients several times a day changing one another's prescriptions!

I was told by the American Hospital Administrator, San Ruohoniemi, that this same German couple had unwittingly saved the hospital from extinction a short while before I arrived. Apparently the hospital had been in dire financial straits. This is not uncommon when the majority of patients cannot afford to contribute to their treatment- of which more later. The only possible solution was to treat foreigners and Nepali paying patients 'privately' and use their fees to subsidise the poor. Robin Hood, Nepal style! As San expressed it "The Lord sent us hippies!" Again, there will be more about hippies and travellers in Chapter 6, but these particular ones were suffering from viral hepatitis resulting from the ingestion of unhygienic food and water on their travels. This condition generally resolves in time, but patients are extremely debilitated for some weeks. (I know this well, because I suffered from it myself a few years later.) To return to my predecessors, though, it seems that standard German treatment at this time was to keep hepatitis patients in bed in hospital for six weeks on intravenous fluids and Dr Peter and Dr Alice were very insistent on this. This potentially developed a good deal of income for the hospital and furthermore the long stay ensured plenty of time to contact their relatives in their own countries (through their embassies) and ensure payment.

Towards the end of Language School, I was summoned to the hospital by the Canadian surgeon, Gordon Mack. It seemed that an official at the Soviet Embassy had acute appendicitis and early surgery was indicated. However, the only anaesthetist, a Nepali, was out of town and no-one else could be located. Would I come and give a spinal anaesthetic? Now anaesthesia was not my specialty and I had never given a spinal. I was reasonably proficient at doing a lumbar puncture, which was the first step, and the surgeon optimistically said: "No problem, you do the LP, inject the stuff and the anaesthetic assistant who has done it loads of times will tilt the patient head up. Bob's your uncle!"

A bit reluctantly, I agreed to this and wished I hadn't when I found that the lady doctor from the Soviet Embassy intended to be present throughout. She turned out to have no English or Nepali and kept signalling to me that I should take the blood pressure! A further complication was that the anaesthetic assistant behind the mask proved later to be a new one and for reasons of his own tilted the patient head down instead of head up. The effect of this was paralysis and loss of sensation from the neck down rather than below the waist. In my innocence, I only grasped this when I started to put a drip in the patient's arm and realised he was not feeling anything! By God's grace, it all worked out well in the end.

Moving to our own house

The time at the guest house was not easy as we tried to balance study with caring for the children who were now interacting with other families and making friends. One new experience came with the visit of the barber, an Indian who would cut our hair in the sunlit garden and try to proceed with the head massage which is a part of all Indian haircuts. I hated it and so did Jamie, who had his first haircut at that time. In his teens, he always grew his hair long; any connection, I wonder? [*Jamie says:* It was so bad that we resorted to a home haircutting kit – which yielded even more lop-sided, ridiculous results.]

Eventually the time came to move to the hospital and to the house nearby. Our boxes and barrels, which we had packed in England nine months before, arrived at the airport from Calcutta at exactly the right time. I went to clear them through Customs, which is always a difficult and confusing task, but I was able to conclude it satisfactorily without having to pay any duty. This was a welcome surprise as we had brought a few electric items that we had thought would be dutiable. Everything got piled on an ancient Indian Tata truck and off we went to the house.

Less satisfactory was the fact that our move coincided with the Winter Rains. While the four month long Summer Monsoon is wet, warm and humid, the winter equivalent is only a few days but wet and cold. The house that the hospital had provided for us lay at the end of a rough path which the rain had turned into a quagmire. It was an unhealthy quagmire at that, since it was used as a latrine for the local people and we dubbed it the Primrose Path. [*Mary says:* Yeah right, see my chapter for what we REALLY called it!] Angela remembers a friend complaining on our behalf to the Director of the Bible and Medical Missionary Fellowship about our living on the Primrose Path, and his reply was "When I was in the army they told you to go out there and get shot and that is what I expect of you". Fair enough!

The house was brick built rather than the traditional mud and thatch or the concrete that became standard in Kathmandu in later years. The hospital had kindly adapted and extended it for use by the incoming family, but this did not run to a Western toilet in the bathroom. Instead, there was an Eastern hole in the floor, but in deference to our peculiar habits, a wooden chair had been constructed with a suitable orifice and this could be placed over the hole in the floor. [*Jamie says (feelingly):* This probably worked better for people who were big enough to actually move it into position!] By the same token, there was neither a bath nor a fitted shower, but an arrangement whereby hot water could be hoisted in a bucket to do service as a shower.

We had taken with us a small Baby Belling electric cooker, but electricity was unreliable, so most cooking was done on kerosene stoves, one of the pressure variety and the other with a simple wick.

The pressure stove was faster and I would use it to make tea when I stumbled down the stairs in the morning. Unfortunately it would often go out, especially as I was leaving the kitchen through the low door, which had not been designed for six footers. As a consequence, on one occasion I turned to go back into the kitchen, forgot to duck and knocked myself out on the doorway.

Angela's comments

We also had a pressure cooker which I used to cook buffalo stew. Initially there was little available other than rice, lentils and an adequate supply of fruit and vegetables in season. I thought at the time that we were really hard done by but by today's standards we could have a healthy diet and one which was good for the figure. During the times we had electricity, which was possibly more than they get it today, cooking on the Baby Belling was fine but the kerosene stoves were nightmares. It was tough.

John again: Enough of these domestic matters—I must go to the hospital.

Chapter 2.

Out of my Depth! First year in the hospital.

As you may remember, I had my fairly new MRCP and thought that made me pretty well qualified. Now I was to find out what it meant to apply that knowledge and those skills in an entirely different arena.

Inpatient work.

I found the wards to be full of relatives! They stayed there, slept the night there and did the cooking for the patients. In the Children's Ward, they even curled up for the night in the cots. These were the "*sathis*", the friends of the patients. One important reason for this was caste, a concept that I had not encountered in practice before. For Hindus their food had to be cooked by a person of the same caste, otherwise they were ritually defiled.

One of my American colleagues found this out the hard way in another context. He was trekking and had high caste porters. They left the meal cooking and went to fetch more water. When they returned to camp, they found him stirring the pot and were aghast. Everything had to be thrown away and the meal started from scratch. This also showed him (and me) our place in the caste system; we are the lowest of all!

The hospital did have a kitchen, but relatively few patients were willing to eat from it. As for special diets, we had excellent dieticians, but they had to be both sensitive and inventive. This was further rendered difficult because of traditional beliefs as to what could and could not be eaten in different conditions. Part of this was *"garmi"* and *"sardi"*. These words can be translated as "hot" and "cold", but actually had little to do with temperature. We were constantly being asked *"Mukh ke ke barnu parcha?"*, or "What things should I avoid eating?" Such advice would mostly be irrelevant, but sometimes it was a good opportunity to advise people to stop smoking or moderate their alcohol intake. In the same way, different concepts of weaning complicated the management of the common malnutrition problems in babies and young children; dieticians and paediatricians alike were constantly struggling with this.

There is a problem about having relatives about all the time; they are eager to speak for the patient, which means it is hard to get the patient's own story, and, having no concept of medical confidentiality, they expect to be told everything. Especially when you are learning a new language, several people speaking at once makes for an impossible situation. I'm afraid I eventually found it essential to ban relatives from ward rounds and outpatient clinics except in special cases.

Touching people was a problem, too. It was recognised that we needed to lay on hands in order to examine a patient, but that was all. I had been accustomed to showing empathy by laying a hand on an arm or putting my arm around the shoulders. However, this too was thought to be defiling and I had to learn not to do it. Even shaking hands was taboo. These caste influences lost their force to some extent in the succeeding years, but were an important factor in those early days.

The range of conditions we saw in the medical wards was entirely different from the ones I had known in England. There was very little chronic arthritis, cardiovascular disease, diabetes, venous thrombosis or asthma and, in those days, very little cancer. This was at least partly because the patients were much younger. Life expectancy then was 42 years for men. Unusually, women's life expectancy was less than their men folk's.

On the other hand, there was plenty of Chronic Obstructive Pulmonary Disease (COPD) which at that time we called Chronic

Bronchitis and Emphysema. I had seen plenty of that at the London Chest Hospital due to cigarette smoking and the tail end of the London smogs, but the epidemiology in Nepal was a bit different. A Nepali colleague later did elegant studies to show that it correlated very closely with the amount of time spent cooking over open wood fires in unventilated rooms and even (inversely) with the size of the rooms. He also showed an additive effect of living at higher altitudes due to reduced availability of oxygen. The result was that we saw many more cases in women than I was used to. Smoking, of course, played its part; the very first industry in Nepal had been a Soviet- built cigarette factory, followed by a match factory.

The biggest difference was the predominance of infectious disease. Most patients were admitted with fever, of which the commonest causes were tuberculosis and typhoid/ paratyphoid fever. Infectious diarrhoeas were common, often amoebic. Amoebic liver abscess, which usually happens without concurrent diarrhoea, was also common. Less common, but still quite frequent were tetanus, rabies and three types of meningitis; tuberculous, bacterial and viral. We saw malaria only occasionally as it does not generally transmit above about 3000 feet in altitude, but we saw it in visitors from the Terai, the lowland part of Nepal, and from India. There were some horrendous cases of septicaemia and it was often not possible to identify the original site of infection. We saw occasional cases of Kala Azar, the Black Fever, due to systemic Leishmaniasis, and elephantiasis due to filarial infection. Of the non-infective conditions, liver failure was common, due to cirrhosis which was often, though not always, alcoholic.

The picture was often complicated by malnutrition (especially in the Children's Ward), worm infestations, scabies and lice.

Elective admissions? There weren't any, even in the surgical wards.

Before even joining the hospital, I had discovered that I could be used as a substitute anaesthetist, but it turned out this was never required of me again. But what else was in store that I hadn't anticipated?

Outpatient work.

I was surprised to find that in Indian and Nepali English this is usually known as "outdoor patients", though not usually conducted *al fresco*. Of course, general physicians (as I was) were accustomed to outpatient clinics, including the assessment and management of patients with diabetes, asthma, COPD, kidney disease and so on, plus follow up of people discharged from the wards. But I was used to working interactively with general practitioners and in those days such people did not exist in Nepal. The hospital was committed to seeing anyone and everyone who came in off the streets and their numbers were huge. We essentially had Surgical, Obstetrics and Gynaecology, Children's and Medical clinics, but the Medical clinic was the one that managed patients that did not fit into the other categories. This meant that it was in many ways like a general practice 'surgery' in the UK. From 8 am, while we were doing our ward rounds, patients would be registering and then waiting patiently to be seen. Noisily, but patiently for the most part! Then we would need to see them all, often a hundred patients for one or two doctors in the Medical Clinic. Meanwhile, we would be responding to emergencies and questions on the wards (I got to know those staircases very well!) and taking turns to see urgent cases in the Emergency Room.

So I found myself general practitioner, dermatologist and emergency physician as well as covering all those things expected of a physician in those days; neurology, gastroenterology, cardiology, respiratory medicine and infectious and tropical disease. At one point, someone even came asking to see Dr Dickinson, whom they had heard of as a psychiatrist!

At one stage, more or less in despair, I sent a message to reception to stop registering patients. This soon brought the Medical Superintendent to my room. "We never turn patients away!" Ouch!

When I mention that I sometimes had a Nepali House Physician (or Intern) working with me, but as often as not was on my own, and that the pattern described was Unrelenting six days a week, you will appreciate that my family did not get to see very much of me in those days. The first year was the worst; the mission expected me to continue language study and to take language exams, so my hours in the hospital were somewhat shortened. (Not by much–I took my language classes at crack of dawn.) As a result, the Medical Superintendent (whom I loved dearly) decreed that I should not be entitled to the day off that other doctors were allowed!

Saturday was the worst day. It is the Hindu holiday, like Sunday for Christians and Friday for Muslims. So, of course, people were off work and free to go to the hospital. The crowds were enormous. Although general outpatient clinics were supposed to be finished in the morning, they often went on well into the afternoon and always did on a Saturday.

Many of the conditions I saw in OPD were reasonably quick to deal with; scabies, bronchitis, urinary infections, diarrhoea, worm infections and so on, though often patients had to be sent to the lab and then come back with the results. Time could be taken up with explanations and advice; smoking, diet, hygiene, water supplies and others. And there was, of course, the bane of the GP's life "While I'm here, doctor..." Many patients had been round the block many times. Shanta Bhawan had quite a good record keeping system and staff to manage it, but the few other Nepali hospitals did not. The same was true of Nepali doctors, often government employees who ran private clinics in their homes or in a small shop. They simply gave everything to the patient; X rays, lab results and scraps of paper on which pre-scriptions had been scribbled. So the itinerant patient would turn up with a large, crumpled roll of these items. There was no appeal in staying with the same doctor or requesting a referral; patients simply went somewhere else if they did not feel better. Some cases were genuinely complicated and some of the patients had been to India or even Thailand for treatment, so they were inevitably time-consuming.

I think there are two kinds of doctor when subjected to this kind of stress. One that I worked with was amazingly patient and method-ical. He treated every patient as if he or she was the only one, taking whatever time was needed. This was great for the patient concerned, but the despair of his colleagues and the waiting hordes. In my case, I was always very conscious of the full waiting room, worked as fast as I could and developed a few tricks. One was to interview a patient whilst another was undressing for examination, and I had a clinic helper who organised that for me. Not so good for confidentiality, but I think it may have been forgiven in the circumstances, if indeed it was noticed. Another was one I've already mentioned with inpatients;

keeping the relatives outside. This was not ideal either and exceptions had to be made. The other thing I did was to organise a proper medical clinic on a different day, one to which I referred patients that I thought would need more time and more detailed consideration. Meanwhile they could get some preliminary tests. Colleagues were able to refer patients to this clinic as well and it gave an opportunity to give some teaching to my House Physician (if I was so lucky as to have one!) In spite of these tricks, I still have a guilty feeling that I was short, brusque or even rude with individuals whilst trying to cope with the masses.

Afternoons were for Private Clinics. At Shanta Bhawan needless to say doctors did not benefit financially, but the fees charged for appointments went into hospital funds to help pay for the treatment of those who could not afford it for themselves. To private appointments came three classes of people, classified by the level of fees. The lowest were Nepalese, Indians and Bangladeshis, next were foreigners from the developed world and at the top were foreigners whose health care was covered by insurance. This may seem unjust, but the foreigners all ended up paying considerably less than they would for equivalent private care in their own countries. In those first few years, we were very popular with the embassies and aid organisations, as there were virtually no other facilities of an equal status.

Not that our advice was invariably accepted; I examined a certain Ambassador on one occasion and strongly advised him to stop smoking and lose weight. His response was "I'd sooner give up doctors!" Amusing at the time, but within a few months he was admitted with a heart attack.

I gave similar advice to a high born young lady from the Rana family. I said that she would have to lose a lot of weight if she was to marry a royal prince like her sisters. I can't think why I was not beheaded!

Emergency Room.

I was relieved not to have to treat children and gynaecology patients in my clinic, but I was required like everyone else to cover the Emergency Room out of hours. This took me into areas in which I had no expertise and increased my feelings of inadequacy. Often it was possible to get another opinion, and I could admit patients under the care of another specialty, but there was not always a specialist available.

My lifetime worst medical memory is of a baby brought in late in the evening allegedly with a 'fever', though the temperature was normal when we measured it. Also he had been seen by another doctor who said he had a heart murmur and needed urgent admission. I could not confirm this and the baby seemed to be normal. Beds were always tight, so I declined to admit him, but arranged for him to be seen by the paediatrician next morning. The parents were not happy with this, but I stuck to my guns. How I wish I hadn't! They brought the baby back about 6 o'clock the next morning and he was obviously very ill. We rushed him to the Children's Ward where he was diagnosed with meningococcal meningitis and died in spite of treatment after a few hours.

There is an interesting sequel to this. The family, a very large one, came from Dhulikhel, a town about 20 miles East of Kathmandu. Later I got to know several of them quite well and felt it right to apologise that I had failed them with the baby. But they never seemed to blame me or feel angry about it. Still later, I taught in a medical school in Dhulikhel and was having a social get together with a group of students on the occasion of my retirement. They wanted to 'interview' me *à la* TV and among the questions was one about my worst experience in medicine in Nepal. So I told them this story, whereupon one of the boys said: "I know that story–he was my brother!" He showed no resentment either. The Nepalese are a joy to know.

Americans!

For the first time in my professional life, I found myself treating Americans. They would be travellers, hippies, aid and embassy personnel and even colleagues in the mission. Of course, they suffered from the same problems as other expatriates such as diarrhoea, hepatitis and dog bites with the dreaded possibility of rabies. But the big difference seemed to me that they were not interested in the possible diagnosis or conclusions that I had come to, but asked "What do the tests show?" They wanted numerical values for their blood counts and chemical tests and exact findings in their stool analysis and I think some even had a reasonable knowledge of normal values, but I had certainly not been used to that.

They often particularly wanted to be treated by an American doctor but we didn't have a clinician from the USA at that time. One lady managed to track down Dr Walter Bond and asked if he would treat her. With his dry sense of humour, he said he was American and willing but pointed out that he was the pathologist and only did autopsies!

They say Britain and America are two countries divided by a common language and I had various experiences of this. It took me a while to learn that the Americans term a doctor like me an "internist", whereas in Britain we generally just say "physician", or at least we did until the proliferation of sub-specialties. I thought I had mastered this subtlety, and I was asked by a member of a visiting American group what sort of doctor I was and answered that I was an internist. She replied- "Oh, so you are not fully qualified yet!" She had understood "intern", which is what junior doctors are commonly called in the USA.

Before I arrived, incidentally, a similar group was apparently asking all the doctors about their specialties. A blunt Australian female paediatrician replied with one word. "Diarrhoea!"

A 'Steep Learning Curve'

My Nepali was improving all the while, but the nurses and my clinic helper had to help me out occasionally. But no-one helped me out on one embarrassing occasion. We had been treating an elderly man for Cor Pulmonale. This occurs when chronic lung disease becomes so bad that the extra strain on the heart causes the heart to fail. Sadly he died and I was trying to explain to the relatives. I meant to say "We gave him lung medicine and heart medicine, but he was too ill to respond". But instead of saying '*mutuko ausadhi*', which is 'heart medicine' I said we gave him '*mrityuko ausadhi*' which means 'death medicine'! They looked shocked and departed and it was only later that I realised what I had said. The politeness of Nepalis is such that none of the doctors and nurses present corrected me.

At the end of a very busy, stressful, but fulfilling year, we went on holiday to Kalimpong which is close to Darjeeling in the hilly, Nepali-speaking part of West Bengal. Darjeeling District, having belonged to Sikkim, was overrun by Nepalese 'Gorkha' soldiers at the beginning of the 19th century. Though British India took it back by treaty in 1815, even now, Nepali is the common language there. We had our first experience of travelling down to the Terai by bus and across the border into India. From there it was a long train journey (on which we celebrated Jamie's 2nd birthday) and then another bus ride up into the foothills of the Himalaya again to Kalimpong. We stayed at a charming old world guest house under the care of a Miss Horgen. It was late September and we had hoped that the monsoon would be giving way to pleasanter conditions, but it was not to be; rain, low clouds and more rain were on the menu. I had hoped (and I am sure Angela had hoped) that I would be able to spend what is nowadays called 'quality time' with the children. I am sad to report that my main memories were of going to sleep and being almost impossible to wake! I remember feeling as if my head was being pressed down into the pillow by an irresistible force.

So ended the toughest year of my life.

Chapter 3.

Mary Poppins in Nepal. By Mary

So. I grew up in Nepal, and I've been asked to tell you all about it. I think it's only fair to warn you at this stage that my budding personality was warped by Mary Poppins. It was like this. I was at the British Primary School in Kathmandu for the first years of my (slightly unusual) education, and every year the school got to go for a Christmas treat to see a film at the British Embassy. This was a major event of the year, films not being something we otherwise had access to. Now the aforementioned embassy only had one film in its library which was considered suitable for vulnerable infant minds, and this was *Mary Poppins.* Most of the kids were with Aid families who only stayed in Nepal a year or two, so this wasn't really a problem. Except for me. I was at this school for six years, and so I saw *Mary Poppins* every year for six years. I know all the words off by heart, even now, when I can barely remember my own telephone number.

Don't get me wrong, it's a great film. But you can't expect to come out of that sort of experience unscathed.

Only in my case the medicine that went down with my spoonful of sugar was Flagyl. The nastiest of all the antibiotics ever invented. It treats a particularly nasty gut bug called Giardia. (You'll recognise it if you ever get it, it gives you egg burps.) My brother Jamie and I always preferred to keep the bug, egg burps and all, and give the

Flagyl a miss, because it only made you feel worse. But my mother fed it to us fanatically. [*Mum says:* WHO considered Kathmandu the unhealthiest city in the world at that time.]

And my father didn't work at the bank, like Jane and Michael's father. He worked at the big mission hospital down the road. In between seeing hordes of patients, he regularly gave *"How to keep healthy in Nepal"* lectures to the newcomers. Only every so often they had to be cancelled because he was sick. [*Dad says:* True, I'm sad to say. The lecture got renamed 'Health Precautions'!]

And when you say "Let's go fly a kite" in Nepal, you don't nip down to the park with a troop of bankers in double-breasted suits decorated with carnations, you trot up to your own flat roof with a supply of unbelievably cheap kites made of brightly coloured tissue paper. You doctor the reel of string with powdered glass and then you try and cut down everyone else's cheap paper kite before they can attack yours. Kites are a competitive sport in Nepal, and don't you forget it.

Magic umbrella would be good

But we digress. A major difference in the real Nepal, the one outside the British Embassy film room, was the travel. Unlike Mary P, I didn't float about gently by umbrella power, or find myself instantly magicked to another world by the snap of my fingers. Trips in Nepal, by bus, plane, elephant, boat, bike, motorbike, *tuk-tuk*, car or hoof, are an experience only for those with a sense of humour. They simply beg to be shared. And perhaps by giving you a flavour of some of these experiences, I can give you an idea of what it was like growing up in Nepal.

Let's start with planes because as I write, I've just booked flights to take my own two kids to visit Nepal for the first time. [See Chapter 17.] The last time I went out was about 18 years ago and even then Kathmandu had changed out of all recognition from the place where I grew up. I remember then standing at the Gatwick departure gate, looking at the green neon sign that heralded my destination, "Kathmandu" and getting delicious tingles and goose bumps. My whole soul sort of soared. Try it; say "Kathmandu" to yourself a few times, doesn't it give you a buzz? No? Oh well, it must just be me.

This time, sadly, there is no direct flight from London any more, and I suspect the sign saying "Doha" and the prospect of a 17 hour trip with 2 kids is unlikely to produce tingles other than of horror.

But then again, perhaps Qatar is less likely to have the kind of landing Royal Nepal Airlines used to achieve when all the gas masks would come down, and you'd be a tad nervous about the rattling of the luggage lockers above you. And nowadays the runway is big enough that planes don't have to slow themselves down with a parachute, and there are so many of them that one landing is no longer a spectator sport for the whole town.

The view will be the same though, and I'll settle for that. Flying into Kathmandu is quite an adventure in itself. The valley nestles at about 4500 feet, surrounded on all sides by foot hills at around 9000 feet, mere pimples on the horizon against the majesty of the Himalayan peaks behind them, but three times the size of our own Ben Nevis. Planes have to enter the valley above these before dropping hastily to land. You arrive to find the time is 5-6 hours and 40 minutes ahead of London, Nepal has its very own individual time zone twenty minutes out from that of India.

[*Dad says:* This has changed! You might expect that Nepal had changed its time zone to one based on differences of whole hours. But no! It was changed by 5 minutes, based on placing Nepal's meridian over the summit of a holy mountain named Gauri Shanker. Nepal Time is now GMT + 5 hours and 45 minutes. This makes for interest, but not for convenience!]

The last time I went (the soul soaring occasion you recall) I queued in a lengthy line to change some travellers cheques for rupees, then queued in another lengthy line for a visa, filled the appropriate form in in triplicate (my brother once wrote "hijacker" under occupation, and nobody ever noticed), only to be told I could only buy my Nepal visa in US dollars. Oddly enough, having flown from the UK, I didn't happen to have any dollars about my person, and I had to trail off to another queue to purchase some. All this time, Dad was waiting for me in some discomfort, having unfortunately been bitten in a very personal place by a stray dog the day before while out jogging. (On the subject of being picked up at the airport, my brother and I remain disappointed to this day that we were never picked up by elephant, which is something that happened to some friends of ours once. You'd think after 6 months in boarding school in India, one's parents would pull out all the stops.)

Anyway I'm rambling. We were talking about planes in Nepal. When I was a child we didn't fly about the place much (there weren't so many planes, and we were too poor) but I do remember a flight down to the Terai (I think Dad got us a freebie there for vaccinating the staff). I remember the cows being chased off the field that was the landing strip, and the plane having to wait until it was clear to land. (I think that time, to be fair, we at least got *to* the airport on an elephant. Or at least I own a picture of Jamie and me patting an elephant's trunk on a field with a plane on.)

What with being poor and all (Don't worry, I'm just bigging that up – we were rich beyond compare in relation to most of the Nepali folk, but my parents got a living allowance rather than a salary and were judged below the poverty line when it came to applying for a grant for my university career) we did a lot of walking. We didn't have a car, though Dad did have a motorbike, which Jamie and I appropriated long before we were old enough to do so. Walking around Kathmandu involves having one eye firmly on where your foot is going. The path to our first house we termed "Oooey Alley" as it appeared to be used as the local toilet. All paths and roads can be used as such by passing children, adults, cows, dogs or elephants, so one treads warily.

And our holiday activity was always trekking. Nowadays, that sounds wonderful to me: days of walking through then unspoiled country (we went to places where people had never seen a white person) with the amazing Himalayas above as if painted by Poppins magic. As a child, however, I am ashamed to confess, I SOO didn't see the point! Why would you walk all day for several days just to get back to the place you started? Why would you sleep in leaking tents or houses on a hard floor, and eat *dal bhat* (which I hated though I love it now) every day for fun? I think the Nepali people agreed with me. On one trek, after asking our destination, and wanting to know all about it, one man looked a bit puzzled, and then broke it to us gently… "Don't you know the bus goes there?!"

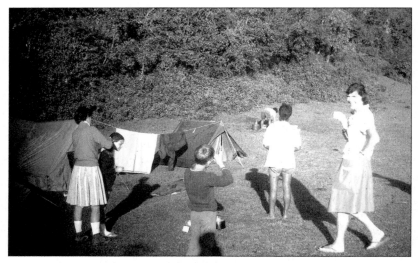

Camping on a trek with school teacher, Ann Lycett

One trek, I sprained my ankle, and Dad took the frame off his ruck-sack and carried me on it, while the porter added Dad's load to his own without any difficulty. [*Dad says:* The ankle was fine next day—I think she was just wanted to be carried!] There's a picture in the family album, I don't know which one of us looks more uncomfortable. When Dad removed the tape he'd strapped my ankle up with, we discovered I was allergic to Elastoplast, and I had to dunk my foot in every river we came to in order to soothe the itch. ("Oh it's a jolly 'olliday with Mary..." Did Dick van Dyke have the worst Cockney accent EVER or what?)

As a family we developed the game of helping my mother over the somewhat precarious bridges she detested. If you've seen *Indiana Jones and the Temple of Doom* and remember the rope bridge high above a gorge where he falls through one of the broken slats, that's pretty much typical. That or the ones that are just a single log optimis-tically placed between one bank and the other in the hope that you can balance your way across without falling off.

Trekking was the only place I've ever liked tea. Instead of being the dishwater-like product we indulge in over here, in Nepal it's spiced and sweet, and gives you the energy to push on through the pain of your blisters up the next several thousand feet of stone steps to the next tea shop. Fortunately there are generally plenty of them.

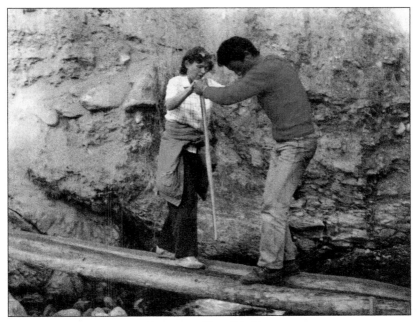

Mum on a Nepali bridge

Jamie and I were teenagers by the time we got to go rafting for a holiday instead. Now THAT was my kind of transport. We had a wonderful trip down the Trisuli River in the early days of rafting. (Though perhaps my clearest recollection of that was trying to force my legs up the all of the 30cm step into the raft. It was the day after we had run round the 30km Kathmandu ring road.) My mother worried about the rapids, and was always asking our guide Krishna if there were rapids round the next bend. To which he would sing out cheerfully "Never know!" which rapidly (pun entirely intended) became a family phrase.

On all these trips, rafting and trekking, and indeed at home, it was family tradition to read a book together. We never had TV, so we had to make our own entertainment with reading and games. When we were smaller, Mum and Dad would take turns reading to us (often Biggles). We'd plead for another chapter... "dear kind most respected father, PLEASE read us another chapter..." be turned down and dispatched off to bed, only to return to say good night to find Dad eagerly reading on.) But later we'd take turns reading Arthur Conan Doyle or John Buchan books to each other, and I remember doing this by candle light in our tent by the river.

Trekking holidays involved lengthy trips in Nepali buses. Think you know what a bus is? Nah, think again. In Nepal, you are crammed in to an old rattling piece of squashed metal on wheels, with all the windows open or broken (open, I'm guessing, so people can vomit out of them or expand out of them if there isn't room on the bus).. There are people in every available bit of air. Nepalese are slight people in the main, so five fit across a four man seat pretty routinely. There aren't just people in the aisles; there are goats and baskets of chickens. There are at least as many people (and animals) along with the luggage up on the roof. These laden, vomit stained Tardises drive along hairpin bends along cliff edges. Their drivers don't really see why you wouldn't overtake on a blind corner. There are no barriers on these roads and buses didn't always stay on them. One of these trips, we came across a landslide completely blocking the road. The driver scratched his head for a bit, then all the passengers, complete with luggage, goats, and chickens, walked over the landslide to a bus in a similar situation on the other side, and both buses turned back and drove back the way they had come. We made it home. We always made it home. Somewhat surprisingly now I think about it. [*Mum says:* There were small Interserve prayer groups in UK praying.]

Talking about holidays and trekking brings Christmas to mind. The best Christmas dinner I have ever had was spam and *chapattis* by a dam on a trek. Grandma used to send us out food parcels of delicacies such as Angel Delight, marmite and spam, and Mum had hoarded the spam to make a special Christmas lunch for our trek. You might not think this sounds special as such, and to be honest I wouldn't touch it with a bargepole nowadays, but trust me, it was the ultimate treat. Not only was trekking fodder continual *dal bhat*, but Christmas lunch most years was partaken in the forest in a huge church gathering. You guessed it—*dal bhat* was eaten from plates made of leaf sewn together with twigs. Being allowed to eat with our fingers (you develop your thumb into a shovel to swoop the hot food into your mouth), the leafy plates, and the antics of the monkeys in the trees; these things slightly made up for it being *dal bhat* and the fact that we'd have to sit listening to an extremely lengthy service that we didn't understand. But in comparison, spam and the peace of the dam was Christmas heaven. (I'm hosting Christmas lunch this year, I wonder if I should put *chapattis* and spam on the menu?)

We were trekking for another Christmas too. This time the porter purchased a chicken to cook along the way, but it escaped and we all found ourselves chasing Christmas dinner along the terraced rice fields. Christmas dinner recaptured, it was later cooked in a beautiful camp site by the side of a river, with an enormous log on the bank providing a blazing camp fire. The porter then produced a cake he'd managed to cook in the campfire. He balanced a solitary fat candle on it to present it to us. It was a happy day.

Back to Kathmandu; once we were old enough, we got around mostly on bikes. Here in England, I insist on walking my 11 year old daughter to school a 10 minute walk away, and I'd be nervous if she went on her own. But I remember clearly at less than her age cycling on my own across the capital city of Kathmandu to go for a sleepover with a friend. (I got a flat tyre, the chain fell off continually, my *chupple* (flip flop) strap broke; it was an eventful journey.)

Traffic in Kathmandu has its own special rules, I recall. Cows have the ultimate right of way on the roads, but after that it's a case of right of way to the biggest vehicle. So on a bike, you have no right of way, and have to stop for every car and truck coming out of the smallest side road. Even now as an adult 40 years later driving on a main road in the UK, my automatic instinct is to stop if I see a truck coming down a side road.

Jamie and I managed to appropriate Dad's motorbike early on. I went along for a driving licence at the age of 14.

"How old are you?" asked the man at the desk.

"14." I said (I'd been brought up by missionary parents.)

"You have to be 16 to drive a motorbike," he said, carefully writing down 16. "Now you have to do a written test."

"But I can't read or write Nepali," I protested.

On hearing this, he cheerfully consigned the written test to the bin, and took me out for the driving part of the test. He carefully explained to me the route I must take on my motorbike. I set off (alone) and when I returned he had gone for a cup of tea and I had passed my test.

[*Jamie says:* OK reader, are you buying this? Licence handed over out of general bonhomie and because my sister was just so lovely? That's not how it works! Everyone knows a few rupees were handed over – you're not fooling anyone sis! (Oh and by the way I may have been, and may continue to be extremely jealous]. [*Dad* denies there was any bribery! But we have always felt Jamie was hard-done-by as he was not allowed a licence at 14.]

After that Jamie and I had many expeditions. The favourite one in family annals is when we'd got into kayaking. This was in the wake of the "Never know" rafting expedition, and an adventure-minded missionary friend and Krishna took us off to some very white water high in the hills kayaking. On that trip, Dad developed the new sport of upside-down underwater kayaking, and learned why you have to wear a helmet as he bounced his head down the rapids. And Jamie literally wrapped his kayak around a large rock. I've never seen him look so pale. Anyway, returning from this trip, we were looking for similar adventure in the Kathmandu valley. Only, of course, by definition, there wasn't a lot of white water around. Fortunately it was monsoon, so the tiny streams that run through the paddy fields had swollen to promising rivers (if you didn't mind the leeches). Our only challenge was how to get the two of us, and the kayak on the motorbike to get to the start. Dad had the sparky notion of purloining the wheels of Mum's old-lady shopping trolley (you know, the ones with a rectangular plaid bag with a handle on a frame with wheels...) It worked a treat. I drove the motorbike (through the cars, rickshaws, bikes, cows, *tuk tuks*, dogs and the usual traffic carnage). Jamie held on to the kayak and pulled it along behind on the wheels of the shopping trolley. Unfortunately the shopping trolley didn't survive, and Mum still holds a grudge.

It was a small 50cc motorbike. [*Jamie says:* It was in fact a monstrous 90cc of sheer brute horsepower. (His latest one was 500cc!)] Such a small motorbike is just not Poppins, and only 2 (plus kayak) can fit (well, two Westerners anyway, a family of 4 on a motorbike is a regular sight in Nepal) so there were other ways we got around our home town of Kathmandu. We could hail a dusty Toyota taxi, or a rickshaw. There was always *a tuk tuk* when I was a child. Or *phutphut* ; I think either describes the noise they make. If you've never been in one of these contraptions, it's like a cross between a moped, a rickshaw, a mini, and one of those orange balloon bouncy things with horns that you hop about on as a child. (Wear a solid bra. Even if you are a man.) And when a trolley bus service was set up between Kathmandu and Bhaktapur, we were regular riders. That *did* seem pretty magical.

But I have to come back to elephants, which perhaps seem the most exotic of my travel options, and must surely set apart my childhood experiences from those of my cousins who grew up in Gerrards Cross. They are (or were) regular features of Kathmandu traffic (the elephants, not my cousins, pay attention!) You would see them hauling loads around the streets, and when we saw the procession for King Birendra's coronation, he was riding high on a grandly decorated elephant. But we got to ride on them when we visited the Terai, the jungle southern part of the country. You bounce along in a howdah on the elephant's back, looking out for wildlife (rhinos and the occasional tiger) and the world is good. The time we were there for the freebie, I had a cold, and we were woken in the middle of the night (along with the tourists who had paid a lot of good hard cash for the privilege of being woken up) to see a tiger (baited with a buffalo calf). Silence was the order of the day (or more strictly, night) in order to see this tiger devouring its prey, but I couldn't stop coughing. The tourists were unimpressed.

When I went on a school trip down to the Terai, our school bus got stuck in the river it had to drive through *en route* home. Two elephants were employed, one to pull and one to push, and we returned to school proudly with a large dent in the ladder at the back of the bus.

I've chosen to structure this chapter around transport, but as I write it, the memories that flood back are those of holidays. Those are the highlights of growing up, and they have to be special to create special memories, and as I write I'm so pleased I've booked that long Qatar flight to take my own children to create their own memories in Nepal.

Was it good for you?

Of course it wasn't all holidays. Too many memories to share, but I remember a yak heart in the fridge when Dad was researching mountain sickness. I remember collecting frogs with him in the pool outside the hospital in the dark by the light of the motorbike head-light for his students' physiology experiment. I remember bargaining for sticky molasses sweets. I remember the long trip across India to visit the boarding school we would be sent to when I was 13. I remember learning to do the Eskimo roll in a kayak in Pokhara lake, and leaving my skin behind in it because we'd got sunburned the day before. I remember getting lost in the caves around the Chobar gorge at the edge of the Kathmandu valley and a search party being set up. I remember dung floors and smoky houses. I remember women and children carrying loads bigger than themselves up steep hills in bare feet. I remember picking off over a hundred leeches in a day. I remember going to the mission hymn "sing song" once a week—well I'm boring you.

It was different, of course it was, but it seemed normal to us at the time. We didn't have sweets and chocolates and TV and grand-parents, and when we were small we missed all of that, and when we did return to England for visits we watched TV continuously (ignoring our grandparents). But I didn't have to get very much older to realise I was very, very lucky to grow up in Nepal. What I did have was breath-taking scenery, an ever-friendly society, adventure and the freedom to develop independence.

I still watch *Mary Poppins* with my kids, but the last time I was at the British Embassy, I'd got all grown up and was visiting Mum and Dad, and *Dick Whittington*, the Christmas panto, was on. It was all "Has anyone seen my Dick?" "Has anyone seen my pussy?" I don't know WHAT Mary P would have thought.

Supercalifragilisticexpialidocious.

Chapter 4.

Second Year and on

The Medical Superintendent
(and some thoughts about abortion!)

Returning to the fray proved a bit more manageable. Now I was allowed a 'day off'. I might well do a ward round and visit the sickest patients again in the evening, but had no clinic duties. So I will start with a word about my early 'boss', Dr Winifred 'Sandy' Anderson. She was certainly a tough Scottish lady of the old school of missionaries, having served many years in India. I've indicated how she expected me to see all the patients registering for my clinic, but she sometimes asked others to help and sometimes they volunteered if their own clinics were not excessive. She was, in fact, the soul of kindness and expected no-one to work harder than she did. You might have expected a long-serving missionary of her generation to be very conservative in her views, but I was amazed at her approach when the question of termination of pregnancy arose. The Nepal government was considering legalising abortions with the very good intention of reducing deaths from the attentions of unqualified 'back street' practitioners. Though I expected her to reject this out of hand, she instituted a series of discussions to see what others thought about it. In the end, it was the Nepali nurses who decided the issue; they would have nothing to do with terminating normal pregnancies! The Nepal Medical Association also had a vigorous debate on the issue. The main contenders against legalising abortion were, strangely enough, the Brahmins (from the priestly high caste) and the few Christian overseas doctors, including myself and Denis Roche from the Bhaktapur Hospital whom I mentioned in Chapter 1.

I'll take the risk of exploring this a bit further, though I know it will be contentious. I deeply sympathise with women who have unwanted pregnancies and fully acknowledge the arguments about back street abortion. I suppose my opposition is not so much because of my Christian beliefs, but my understanding of biology. It is really impossible to identify the point at which an embryo or foetus becomes human, except at the point of conception when the genetic elements of the two parents come together to make a new individual. So, to me, destroying a foetus is no different from destroying a new born baby, or indeed an adult. I know this will seem hard to some folk, but it seems to me the correct ethical position if we are not to weaken the principle of the sanctity of human life, which is dear to people of most religions and to humanists.

In the end, the government dropped the idea, though abortion was legalised under certain conditions many years later. In the meantime, women were sent to prison for having abortions while the men who got them pregnant went scot free and I hated the injustice of this.

Sandy was the obstetrician and gynaecologist and came to retirement in my second year. She was replaced as obstetrician by Mary Eldridge, a lady who had taught me obstetrics in medical school and who was much loved by patients and colleagues alike for her professionalism and caring nature.

Surgeons

I worked with a series of interesting surgeons, though I can't mention them all. Gordon Mack was a Canadian with high professional standards and no real interest in learning Nepali. In spite of that, he gained a high reputation among the surgical fraternity in Nepal. He was replaced by a gentle, patient, caring Canadian called Gerry Hankins who became a really close friend and colleague as well as a cross country running companion. Later came Dick Matern, a dedicated, rather eccentric American surgeon. He and his wife and daughter lived above us for a while and we had great amusement watching him trying to teach an orphaned baby owl to fly. He stood below the balcony while the others held the owl on top, calling "Come to Mother, Herky!" Didn't work! Another overheard call was when he was off to operate on yet another emergency; "I'm going to the OR (Operating Room) and I'll be there till the Pope gets married!"

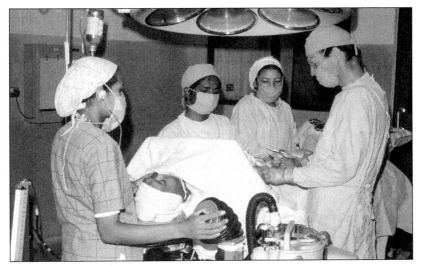

Surgery at Shanta Bhawan Hospital. Photo: Dr Gerry Hankins

Paediatrician

Liane Nitschke was our German Paediatrician. She was energetic and full of compassion and, though her English was good, she had some interesting and charming variations. "Zis child is very much malnutrished" was a favourite of mine and though I teased her sometimes I could hardly criticise as I don't have more than a few words of German. She waged war on intestinal parasites in her young patients, including the roundworm, Ascaris lumbricoides. I am sure I once heard her declaiming "I am ze great enema of ze Ascaris!" With her big heart and determination, though a single lady, she adopted and brought up an orphaned baby Nepali girl in Nepal and later in Germany.

Pathologist

I have mentioned Walter Bond, our American pathologist with his dry sense of humour. He was responsible for all the laboratory services and performed the autopsies. These were usually on expatriates as the Nepalese were reluctant to give consent for post mortem examinations, wanting to take the bodies of deceased relatives to the river *ghat* as soon after the death as possible. Later on, the government and police made autopsy obligatory for some cases, but only Nepali doctors were permitted to perform them. They were often not well trained and I actually saw one of them standing masked and gowned at the opposite end of the post mortem room making notes while a '*peon*' (errand boy) actually made the incisions in the corpse. I greatly valued Walter's meticulous autopsy reports when I was doing the research on Acute Mountain Sickness which I will recount later.

There was an American lady who was responsible for the hospital guest house. This had been the gambling den in the old Rana palace and stood in the charming Butterfly Garden. Visiting mission folk and others stayed there in comfort for a reasonable cost, but anyone who was able to afford to go on the very expensive Mount Everest tourist flight was charged a great deal more.

I have begun with some expatriates, but many of my favourite colleagues were the Nepalese. PB Rai was an ex-Gurkha soldier who signed up for the Army at the illegally early age of 16. "I was always a big lad!" He had worked in the operating room, but following an illness he was put in charge of the outpatient department and did a great job for many years. His wife, Ringey, was a ward sister and later a nursing supervisor. She had been a Buddhist, but was never reluctant to interrupt my ward round to tell a patient how she had become a Christian.

Nurses

The nurses generally were a delight. They were mostly young and looked lovely in their white saris. (With all due respect to Muslims, I'm so thankful to have been called to a country where women don't wear veils!) Their cheerfulness and willingness made up for their limited understanding of disease processes. They would always do exactly as they were told, though it was usually best to write it down as they didn't necessarily understand the instructions and were too polite to ask for a repeat.

I sometimes asked the nurses for a translation with patients whose first language was Newari, especially the women who often had no Nepali. On one occasion I thought, mistakenly, that the nurse with me was a Newar. Initially she looked blank, but then ran the length of the ward to bring a Newari-speaking nurse.

Though many of the 'nurses' on the ward were still students, they played a full part in patient care, including night duty, and made a big contribution. We had our own nursing school and I enjoyed giving classes there, but it was at the practical nursing that they excelled. Later regulation of nursing training led to higher academic standards (not necessarily in related subjects) and a decline in the amount of time doing the important practical things. As a result, we used to have to give them extra practical training after they had qualified and joined the staff. Sometimes 'progress' is not progress!)

They had some curious expressions. "The patient is gasping" meant that the patient was thought to be dying. "*Ex bhayo*" meant the patient had become "ex", ie had died! They preferred "expired" to "died".

Nepali doesn't have definite and indefinite articles, so 'one' may be used to indicate a particular person or object. On occasions when the staff used English (which were not often) I would get called from outpatients with "Doctor, you have one patient". I usually managed to resist screaming "Look, I have hundreds!"

Money Matters

Before introducing more colleagues, I need to talk about the difficult matter of money. Even the simplest medical care is expensive; medicines, supplies, bandages, dressings, surgical instruments, water, electricity, rubbish removal and maintenance are just a few of the costs of running a hospital. A large proportion of hospital outlay is the payment of salaries. Also, though we were in no position to offer pensions, we did run a provident scheme to help staff with the expense of buying or repairing a house. Of course, it would be delightful to treat every single patient free of charge without anxieties about funding it, but it can't happen. People in our sending countries were certainly generous, and often it was possible to raise money for capital equipment such as X-Ray or operating theatre equipment, but such sources can never cover the cost of running expenses. Even today, in the tax-funded UK NHS, we see hospitals having major problems meeting their budgets. In the USA there are major controversies about the right way to meet health expenses. How much more in a mission hospital in Nepal in the late 1960s-70s?

Enter the Social Service Department! Our colleague, Shirley Snell (who later became engaged to be married to a mission engineer, Martyn Thomas, while house-sitting in our house) was a fully trained social worker. However she used to say that the work of her department was the work of an old-fashioned almoner; determining who can and must pay for their treatment and who was to receive 'charity' in the form of free treatment or reduced bills.

Sensibly, Shirley did not make these assessments herself; she had Nepali colleagues who would take a detailed history of patients' circumstances. How many buffalo did they have? How many chickens? How many acres of land? What responsibilities? What effect would paying for medical care have upon their lives? They needed the Wisdom of Solomon. Some people who were very poor would try to conceal their poverty out of shame, or, alternatively, pride. On the other hand, those with adequate means would try to get their treatment free, for example by coming to the hospital in old clothes and removing wrist watches, jewellery or other evidence of prosperity.

Bir Bahadur Khawas carried a lot of this load of responsibility. As a Christian from Kalimpong in the Darjeeling District of India, he was much less susceptible to pressure or bribery from local people. He was, in any case, a man of high integrity. The son of a lowly worker in Kalimpong, he had trained as a carpenter before joining the hospital staff. As time went by, he became more and more trusted and respected, became an assistant to the hospital administrator, then the head of the administration. After the move to Patan Hospital in 1982, he was one of the three Officers of the Hospital and then was appointed as Chief Executive of the Hospital after I ended my spell as Hospital Director in 1986.

In Social Services, he was succeeded by Chhogen Rongong who was also a man of high integrity. One could always detect the strain that these men carried as they made scores of difficult judgements every day. As doctors, we might occasionally clarify a point or two, but we would never try to influence their decisions or question their judgements.

Coming back to Administrative Officers, the first one I encountered at Shanta Bhawan Hospital was an American of Finnish origin called Sanfrid Ruohoniemi. He was very capable and active, but sadly, a few years later, he was under my care with recurrent malignant melanoma, a very dangerous form of skin cancer. He developed seizures from deposits in his brain and I could do no more than be with him when he died. Almost simultaneously, two of our colleagues, one Dutch and the other American, were being married in a nearby garden. Sadness and joy on the same day! In a way, this symbolised for me the intensity of the lives we were living in those days.

The relationship between the Administrative Officer and the doctors has an inherent tension. Our task is to treat the patients; his (or hers) is to balance the budget. When I had worked under the NHS in the UK, I had no need to worry personally about the cost of the treatment I was giving, but these concerns are inevitable in a charitable institution like a mission hospital. So I had to consider these things in the context of each patient, just as the heroes in the Social Service Department had to do with those who were referred to them.

Clearly it was necessary to use the most economical effective treatment for each patient. Sometimes we needed to opt for economy at the expense of a degree of effectiveness. I will come back to tuberculosis (TB) later, but we had large numbers of TB patients. At that time, the standard treatment was reasonably inexpensive, streptomycin, isoniazid and thiacetazone. However patients' bacteria would sometimes become resistant to those drugs or they would suffer serious adverse effects. The alternative drugs were extremely expensive, and again and again I found myself in the position of being unable to give treatment that might have a good chance of success.

The same considerations influenced the plans made for the development of the hospital. When I joined, such policy matters were too weighty for the likes of me, but I knew there had been a move to declare the hospital a "Centre of Medical Excellence". This was never acted upon and in retrospect I think that was certainly the right decision. I believe it would have led to the development of increasingly specialised departments offering more and more sophisticated treatment which would have been beyond the means of patients and of those who supported the hospital. True, there would have been an increase in the "private" income that I have described, but one could not help feeling that the poor and needy would have been squeezed out. Later in its history, Nepal developed a large number of private hospitals, but the purpose that had drawn us to Nepal was not private practice. Good basic care was our priority and it was no good aspiring to do Nepal's first heart transplant

Our Nepali Staff

I am glad to say, our staff were loyal, worked hard and gave good service to the patients. Compared to employees in the government hospitals, they worked longer hours, but were paid more in salary and benefits. They knew what was expected of them and cooperated fully, coming to work on time, taking only reasonable tea and meal breaks and not leaving early when there was work to be done. They seemed to take pride in working in an organisation that functioned efficiently and gave good health care in spite of great pressures of numbers.

One thing surprised me early on, and I suppose it was a cultural thing. His Majesty King Mahendra Bir Bikram Shah Dev died on 31 January 1972 of a heart attack during a tiger hunting trip in the Terai, the flat part of Nepal bordering India. He was only 52 years old and it was quite a shock to the nation. The nation generally responded to the news by shutting down in order to mourn. This is not unusual, but I, at least, was surprised that it extended to the hospital staff. I would have thought that they were delivering essential services and that the best tribute to His Majesty would be to continue serving his subjects in need of care. My view was obviously not the prevailing one!

It was several years before the hospital work was threatened again. This time it was industrial action and it came out of the blue. Incited by groups doing similar things elsewhere, the hospital staff suddenly declared a strike. Though many did not join in, especially the doctors and nurses and the expatriates, it was hard to keep patient care going. I have a clear memory of one of the junior Nepali doctors scrubbing the floor of the children's ward because the cleaners were on strike. This was particularly creditable bearing in mind the caste structure and the very hierarchical nature of Nepalese society. We all took on tasks beyond our usual roles. After the strike had begun, the staff representatives (were they really representative?) submitted a list of 30-odd demands that had to be met before they would return to work. The administration had never seen any of these demands before and some were easily met, such as extra blankets for the beds of the student nurses.

Most of the jobs were too much in demand for this to go on very long, and the administration of the time managed it all very tactfully. Though things appeared to return to normal, mutual trust took some time to restore.

Chapter 5.

TB Tales

I t was not my usual barber's shop but it was quite near the hospital. As I chatted away with the skinny barber I felt constrained to comment on his cough. Yes, he had had it some years and it was getting worse. Some further informal history taking revealed that he had taken treatment, including daily injections, but had stopped it as soon as he felt better. He had been back to the doctors several times and had further treatment, though not for very long at a time, and had finally been told that the drugs were no longer working and no more could be done.

It was obvious that the blasts of tussive air that were being sprayed around my neck and ears contained an aerosol of resistant acid fast TB bacilli. Fortunately for me, the resistant organisms are thought to be rather less virulent than their sensitive relations and my initial BCG-induced immunity had doubtless been topped up by frequent exposure.

The Problem of TB

The problem of TB is a huge one in developing countries. Not only are crowded conditions and malnutrition conducive to its spread, but there are many social, geographical and financial factors that make it hard to persuade patients to complete a full course of treatment

My mentor, Denis Roche, was a great warrior in the fight against TB. He would say "The treatment of TB is streptomycin, isoniazid, thiacetazone and *'gali'*. Now *'gali'* properly means a good ticking off and that is what he gave patients who were irregular in their treatment. But he was really a very gentle soul and I'm sure that nowadays he would have chosen a more politically correct expression like 'patient education'. He taught me always to impress on TB patients from the very beginning that it was important to continue on treatment for 18 months and to attend for regular reviews and repeat prescriptions.

It was usually possible to discontinue the streptomycin injections after 2-3 months and continue on oral treatment. Whilst having the injections, patients would need to attend some kind of clinic daily. This was not easy to do, as they may have lived a long way from a suitable facility. Often they would need to stay in or near the hospital with all the disruption to their employment, farm or domestic duties. In most cases, they were feeling much better by the end of this time and needed less frequent visits. It was then that they questioned the need for further treatment and all too often defaulted from treatment.

This problem with default from treatment is all to do with resistance of the TB bacteria to the drugs. The organisms cause chronic rather than acute disease and they have the ability to live for many years in a dormant state deep in the host's cells. They can then awaken and cause more trouble, either in the short term of a few months or later in life, for example when immunity decays due to age or when it is impaired by other factors, nowadays predominantly HIV infection, but also diabetes, or treatment with steroids for another condition. (The HIV/AIDS epidemic was only detected in 1981 and probably did not exist as a human condition much before that. Nowadays, it is a potent cause of the failure to control TB)

So incomplete treatment would result in relapse, but, even worse, the bacteria could become resistant to the standard drugs when the treatment was inadequate. In the days of which I write, there was no possibility of treatment of resistant TB with rifampicin, ethambutol or pyrazinamide because they were just too expensive for all but the wealthiest. Drug resistant TB was a disaster for public health, but also for individuals as my next story will show.

Saila's Father

"Saila" is not so much a name as a status; the third son in a family. [*Jamie says:* the names keep going fourth oldest, fifth oldest …. down to youngest and then something like SURPRISE! Or possibly ACCIDENT!] This particular Saila was a close friend of my own family, though in some sense he was also an employee as he acted as paid porter, guide and cook on our treks in the Himalaya. He would stay in our house when in Kathmandu and we sometimes visited his village, a day's bus ride plus a day's walk away. In fact he said we were the first Westerners to visit it, though there had been one Japanese. I can well believe this because an old woman seeing me for the first time asked where the new Brahmin had come from! On one occasion, Jamie attended Saila's brother's wedding and acted as official photographer. He had the only camera! [*Jamie says:* I also learnt about *chang* (beer) and *rakshi* (moonshine) in the process.]

You will see that the families knew each other well, we communicated very satisfactorily and there was mutual trust. When Saila's father got TB he initially went to a local clinic but soon defaulted from treatment. When the inevitable relapse occurred Saila brought him to me. As he responded to treatment quite quickly I was encouraged to think that his organisms were still sensitive. I emphasised repeatedly, both at the hospital and every time we met, that he must continue to the end of the course and I really thought they had taken the message on board. However after a few months he defaulted again.

Because of his farming commitments, I had no opportunity to raise the matter with Saila. The next I saw of his father was when he was brought to the hospital *in extremis*. Because the hospital treatment had 'failed' he had spent a lot of money on the *jhankri,* a type of traditional healer. We did what we could but there was no hope of success. Saila was heartbroken. I went in search of him in the bazaar and eventually found him in the vegetable market. There I sat on the curb and held him in my arms as the strong man sobbed like a baby. We have the weapons with which to overcome this disease, but so often it is not enough.

Unfortunately, in the early 1970s, the government of the time decided to close the mission hospital near Bhaktapur where I had served my apprenticeship with Denis Roche. (It became a Nepal Army barracks.) The new, replacement, hospital in the town had not been built, so the services that the mission hospital had been providing were completely lost for some years. One of these was the TB detection and prevention service. Ganga Basnet was a young man who had been successfully treated for TB and Denis had trained him to visit homes in villages and in the town to follow up patients on treatment and to detect new cases. Ganga was a powerful asset in preventing relapse and drug resistance. I am glad to say that Denis joined us at Shanta Bhawan for a while and became a great help to the TB clinic among other things. We were also able to employ Ganga in a similar role to the one he had played in Bhaktapur District and he did a good job for many years.

Many years later, Denis and family moved back to Droitwich and he was employed as a Public Health Officer in Worcestershire. On one occasion, I asked him what this involved and, in his usual self- deprecating way, he said: "I do Ganga's job".

Chapter 6.

Hippies and travellers

Hearing a sudden cry for help from the nurses, Dr Dick Matern and I set off towards the hospital gate in hot pursuit of a naked young white man making a dash for freedom. Shanta Bhawan was anything but a prison, but occasionally young travelling westerners were a danger to both themselves and to others. After a brief struggle, in which Dick's only pair of spectacles got broken, we were able to pacify him and return him to the safety of the ward. The crowd of astonished Nepalis gradually dispersed.

In the 1960s and 70s, Nepal was a Mecca for hippies and other young people. Why did they come? Probably for adventure as young people have always done, sometimes as a deliberate rejection of the lifestyle of their own parents and their own countries, sometimes the avoidance or delay of taking up responsibilities. In many cases it was the pursuit of drugs and in others a quite deliberate desire to seek and learn about religions such as Hinduism and especially Buddhism.

They often came overland through Central Asia, in old vehicles or on buses. Nepal was ideal for them. Living was cheap and addictive drugs were openly available in the bazaar. "Get your hash here!" was commonly seen outside shops in Kathmandu. Monasteries opened their doors to disciples from Western countries, some quite genuinely welcoming seekers, others very cynically exploiting them. I heard of monasteries where young travellers were charged large sums of money but, in the name of asceticism, were provided with cramped living space and minimal food. They were encouraged to spend long periods fasting and meditating, with often dangerous results.

Diseases in Travellers

These young people came to us for the treatment of a wide variety of overlapping physical and mental conditions and I will try to explain the background as I understood it.

Nutrition.

Nepalese, at least in the hills, live on *bhat* or rice. (Terai dwellers eat bread instead, usually *chapattis*.) You are not asked if you have had a meal, you are asked if you have eaten rice. They can eat huge platefuls of it, providing a lot of energy and a certain amount of protein and vitamins. Almost invariably, they add *daal*, a thick lentil soup. Nepalis often say they have two meals a day; in the morning rice and *daal* and in the evening *daal* and rice. They will also have some curried vegetables and will add some meat if they can afford it, in many cases only on rare occasions. (Members of the higher Hindu castes may well be vegetarian on principle.) In this way, they may get an adequate diet, though protein may be insufficient. But travellers and other expatriates can rarely manage the large quantities of rice required and, especially on a limited budget, may become relatively malnourished.

Infectious Disease

As well as the nutrition issue, a major problem for travellers was that the Nepal environment contains an army of bacteria, viruses and parasites to which, at least to some extent, the Nepalese have become immune during their childhood. If they have not acquired immunity, they have probably died as a result of infection. I'm talking now about E.coli, Salmonella, Shigella, Campylobacter and the many bacterial causes of dehydrating diarrhoea and dysentery, plus parasites such as Giardia and Amoeba and some viruses. All these spread freely through food and water and the water system in Kathmandu was well and truly contaminated. Though some attempt was made to chlorinate the drinking water at reservoir level, there was constant flow of ground water into the distributing system, especially as farmers needing water for irrigation would simply break into the drinking water pipes. Travellers did not have the same level of immunity and therefore diarrhoea was a constant problem, sapping their strength and contributing to their malnutrition.

Another water- borne infection that wrought havoc among visitors was infectious hepatitis due to the Hepatitis A virus. I have mentioned this before; a very debilitating condition that lasts 6 weeks or more.

Mental Problems

On top of these physical problems were mental ones. I have always thought that at least some of the psychotic conditions we saw had existed from before the travels began and that a certain mental instability had been a reason for the young person detaching him-or herself from the family, perhaps following misunderstandings and rows. But their lifestyle in Nepal was also a risk factor for poor mental health; drugs, including hashish, are known to predispose to psychosis and, of course lead to feelings of unreality. Buddha taught that all life is illusion; nothing is real. Behind much meditation, fuelled by fasting and perhaps drugs, is the desire to 'transcend' reality and free oneself from the fetters of rational thought. It always seemed to me that this was a recipe for a mental catastrophe and a reason why we had a steady stream of disturbed young westerners coming under our care.

I was not a psychiatrist and there were strict limitations to what I could do. In the case of a real psychotic crisis, I would forcibly sedate such people and keep them at least mildly sedated whilst working out what to do. There are a lot of ethical issues involved in this, such as consent, patient autonomy and a patient's capacity to make decisions for him- or herself. The 'bottom line' was the need to act in the patient's best interests according to my best judgement, given that these patients temporarily did not have the capacity (in our opinion) to make decisions for themselves. There was no Mental Health Act to guide me. There was none to protect me, either, but on the other hand no legal mechanism to act against me if I got it wrong. It was a lot of responsibility to take on one's shoulders in one's early 30s!

I could not undertake psychiatric treatment on a long term basis and the main object was to get these folk back to their own countries and families as soon as possible. For this, we needed to enlist the help of the relevant embassy and I got to know the consular departments quite well. They had better communications with their countries than we did and could often make connection with parents or other responsible persons. My experience was that parents generally were ready to take responsibility for at least the costs of treatment and repatriation. I don't know if this arose out of family ties or guilt or any other emotion, but certainly the Embassies, without exception, refused to have anything to do with repatriation unless the costs were guaranteed.

Repatriations!

Though there was very often a degree of improvement in the mental state after some days of sedation and my crude psychiatric treatment, it very often became necessary to provide a medical escort for the repatriation process. My patient; my job! I have to say that I sometimes welcomed the break from routine and the relentless pressure of work, but this would be tempered by the fact that my colleagues would have to cover for me whilst managing their own responsibilities. (I hate to use the term 'workload' because we regarded it as a privilege to serve everyone who came, but the pressures were, in fact, enormous.)

My first experience of this was during my first monsoon season in Nepal. The patient was a young, psychotic Uruguayan man and I had visions of accompanying him all the way to South America. Fortunately, we were able to get authority to accompany him to New Delhi, where there was a Uruguayan embassy, and deliver him into the care of an Indian psychiatrist.

The nurses found him an ill-matched selection of clothes for the journey, but unfortunately could not come up with any shoes. I doubt if he had worn shoes for a while anyway, so it didn't seem to matter; until we came down the aircraft ramp onto the hot tarmac of Palaam Airport! There was a shriek and he promptly punched me! I guess I deserved it for not having anticipated this particular complication, but somehow it had not been part of my training!

The Indian psychiatrist did not appear very interested in the patient, apart from despatching him to his unit. This particular Indian turned out to be an ardent Anglophile; one of those who believe that the worst thing to happen to India was that the British left. Accordingly, he insisted on escorting me to the hotel that had been arranged by the Uruguayan embassy. (Incidentally, I didn't meet any Uruguayans.) He then took me to dinner and then drove me around Delhi on a private historical and cultural tour. Next day I returned to Nepal after what had been a very brief but in some ways enjoyable 'holiday'.

To digress a bit, on the return flight, bad weather caused us to be diverted to Bhairawa in the Terai and land there. On the ground, I got talking to the pilot and asked how they managed to find the Kathmandu Valley through the monsoon clouds. He said: "When we are airborne, come onto the flight deck and I will show you".

So I did, and expected to be shown a radar system or something else highly technical. Instead of that, he indicated a pointed hill ahead and said: "We go there and turn left!"

After the turn, things got a bit tense until the co-pilot suddenly Said: "There it is" and pointed to a gap in the clouds through the right hand window.

The pilot said: "You take it" and the co-pilot dived us down through the clouds to emerge in the Valley. They then proceeded to land the aircraft with me standing between them on the flight deck.

Further trips involved escorting patients to the UK and the Netherlands. After I had handed over the first of these to a doctor at Heathrow Airport, I tried to contact my parents. The first problem was that, while I had been in Nepal, the UK had changed from the old pounds, shillings and pence to metric currency, so, in my tired after-journey state, I had to struggle to identify the coins to put in the pay phone. Then, as it happened, my parents were out, so I phoned my sister and said "This is John" to which came the puzzled reply "Which John?" Anyway I was eventually re-united with my family which was a pleasant bonus.

On one trip, I was recovering from infectious hepatitis myself, was still jaundiced and probably looked worse than the patient. On another, we were on a Pan American flight from Delhi to Europe when the American pilot gave us an update on our position. "Ladies and Gennlemen, we are passing over the border of Pakistan and….

Pakistan and…. Well, we are passing over the border of Pakistan!" Not designed to instil confidence!

One female patient was particularly disturbed and I felt that I would need to sedate her with injections on the flight. I was not hopeful about finding a vein while sitting in an aircraft seat, so I pre-positioned a cannula in the back of her hand. Then it seemed to me she would probably pull it out, so I encased both her hands in plaster of Paris and bandaged them together. This looked dramatic and, I think, might have got her some sympathy from the other passengers. That is, until we were on the ground at Istanbul and she started screaming "Get me off this plane!" Another injection—quickly!

I learned to carry a letter of authority from the embassy or, failing that, the hospital. This followed an account from a Peace Corps doctor who had accompanied a patient to the USA via Heathrow. During transit to another flight, the patient approached a security officer and claimed that he was being kidnapped by a man impersonating a Peace Corps doctor! Apparently it took a while to sort that one out.

Some serious inpatients

Coming to serious physical conditions in travellers, I was sad to treat a young Dutch woman for poliomyelitis, which was already becoming rare due to immunisations. According to her own story, she had been advised by the Dutch authorities not to be immunised, but I can't verify that or, if true, understand it. She was on her honeymoon, and became quite seriously paralysed. Much of the paralysis persisted and she eventually had to use a wheelchair. I met her when she was visiting in Nepal many years later and was further saddened to hear that she was divorced from her husband, presumably because of her disability. However she did seem to have come to terms with the adversity in a quite admirable way.

As a Christian and a mission doctor, I believe in the power of prayer; of course I do! But the next story reinforced my belief that we should also give responsible treatment in addition to praying for, and with, our patients. A young couple had been travelling in Assam. In this instance, I don't think they were married. The man developed a fever and was admitted to my ward, though unfortunately I was away on one of those escorting trips. One of my colleagues was covering for me; excellent in his own field, but that was surgery. Because the man was jaundiced, it was thought that he had hepatitis. If I had been there, I would have questioned that, because it had been my experience that fever, although it occurs in the early stages of hepatitis, has usually gone by the time jaundice is apparent. This patient had a high fever as well as jaundice. When I returned, I found him very seriously ill and with a persisting high fever. I immediately requested blood smears for malaria and he proved to have a very high parasite count in his red blood cells. The parasite was Plasmodium falciparum, the worst of the malaria parasites and the most likely to be fatal. We treated him urgently, but could not save him; he died soon after.

However, that was not the end of this tragic story. Sometime later, his girlfriend was also admitted with high fever and was extremely ill. We barely had time to confirm that she also had falciparum malaria before she died. Of course, we had advised her to come at once to the hospital if she developed any fever, but it transpired that she had been staying with a Christian Scientist couple who had advised her not to go to a doctor. They would pray for her and she would be fine. This went on for several days until they finally panicked as her condition worsened and brought her to hospital; too late.

The strange tale of 'Josh'

The next story is a most extraordinary one about a young man who had a chaotic history and caused me a great deal of trouble. Yet it had a happy outcome and we became good friends. Bearing in mind the slight risk that he might be recognisable, I'm going to call him Josh, though it isn't his name. Josh was a Jewish American who gravitated to Nepal seeking to study Buddhism. I forget why he first came to the hospital; it may even have been an episode of self- harm. He later got admitted to the surgical ward with an ulcer on his toe. This should have healed quite quickly in a young man, but it didn't and various medical explanations were sought. It turned out we were looking in quite the wrong direction. He was finally found dipping his foot into one of the ground level Asian toilets and repeatedly re-infecting the ulcer! Was this evidence of mental illness? Again, there was a different explanation; he had fallen madly in love with one of our Nepali nurses! Not being able to bear being parted from her, he found a novel way of staying in the ward.

Not long after, Josh was discharged from hospital and actually married his lady love in a Hindu ceremony, though I am sure her family were not at all pleased. Unsurprisingly, it didn't work out in the long term; he remained quite unstable. A divorce ensued, though perhaps it was simply recognition that the marriage was not valid in the first place. I don't know as I wasn't involved at that point. Various people helped him at this time, including an international group of young people and a social worker at Shanta Bhawan. As a result, he became a Christian. Years later, he told me that I had played a part in this, which mystified me. According to his account, he had heard me singing hymns as I cycled up the hill to the hospital. (We were in a different house by this time.) I found that hard to believe; I didn't remember doing it and doubted if I would have had the breath!

Angela remembers, though I don't, that he came to and enjoyed one of our Christmas Day parties. These were hilarious affairs with Nepalis and people from lots of other nations, each being required to entertain us or introduce a game. I think it was Gerry Hankins and his family who taught us a game that involved winking, something the Nepalis had never even heard of! They got the idea, but only with much facial contortion, giggling and amusement.

She also recalled going with Josh to a midnight Christmas communion—the first he had attended after he became a Christian. I must have been on duty that night (or perhaps in need of catching up on sleep!)

I think his next move was to join a Protestant Christian community in Amsterdam, but he was not done with his travels. He joined the Roman Catholic Church for a time, but left that to go to Israel as a Messianic Jew (a Christian Jew). There he was happy at first; living on a kibbutz. Then he found that he was required to do the mandatory military service. So off he went again!

As far as I know, his next and final stop was in another Asian country, which I will not name as he is still there. In that country he made a living as a teacher of English, married a local Christian girl and between them they brought up a daughter who was quite severely crippled from an early age. This was not easy for them as the disabled are rather poorly tolerated in that particular country.

At one point, Josh dictated his entire life story on a tape, which he posted to me. He had clearly become a stable, happily-married husband and father with a settled Christian faith. People use the expression 'spiritual journey' but there can rarely have been one as tortuous as this. Jew–Buddhist–Hindu- Protestant–Catholic and Protestant again. Who can doubt that God moves in mysterious ways?

Hepatitis

Adult Nepalese generally don't get hepatitis; they have acquired the infection in childhood, when it is usually mild or even unnoticed. Even my own children had it mildly; I'm afraid I told my daughter to stop fussing and threw her into a swimming pool before I noticed that she was jaundiced! [*Mary says:* Caring father right?! (To be fair as my main symptom of hepatitis was not feeling like swimming, I think I got off rather more lightly than Dad did!)]

I have mentioned treating a lot of travellers for hepatitis, and I certainly didn't keep them in bed for six weeks on IV fluids like my predecessors. I also managed to contract the infection myself and spent a week or two in bed, sick as a dog, eating very little and with no energy at all. Our kind Australian Nursing Superintendent brought me ice cream; a great treat and the envy of the children. I thought I had recovered, but discovered that it was not so when I kept a date for a game of tennis with the Military Attaché at the Soviet embassy–and lost!

Diarrhoea

There was a strong tendency for any conversation among expatriates in Nepal to turn towards diarrhoea and dysentery! To some extent it could be avoided by shunning raw foods, salads and anything that had been exposed to flies before being sold or in the kitchen. Also it was necessary to drink only treated water and boiled milk. One Everest expedition was asked how they handled the problem of drinking water in Nepal and explained that they filtered the water, boiled it, treated it with iodine, then threw it away and drank beer! In the case of our adult wards, we were generally most likely to have diarrhoea patients who were travellers, then expatriate residents

66

and least likely Nepalese. Incidentally dysentery, contrary to general usage, technically just means 'diarrhoea with blood'. As most forms of diarrhoeal disease resolve spontaneously with time, the therapeutic challenge was to treat or avoid dehydration and resulting shock, which is the complication that can kill patients.

In outpatients, we were overwhelmed by travellers with diarrhoeal disease not severe enough to warrant admission. It was cumbersome; after registering and paying the small registration charge, they would wait to see me. Then I would interview and examine them in the busy general clinic. Then they would have to go, via the cashiers' long queue, to produce a stool sample that was examined in the lab for cells, ova and parasites. Next they would have to return to me with the result so that I could prescribe the correct treatment. Then they would have to visit the cashiers again and finally the pharmacy for medicines. So I introduced a more streamlined 'Travellers' Diarrhoea Service'. They paid for the stool test on registration, then went to get it done and came to see me with the result. This saved time for everyone. There was some hilarity at this idea among my colleagues, especially with Americans who thought it amusing to have a diarrhoea service run by someone called John! [For those who don't know, 'the John' is an Americanism for the toilet!] In fact some 'friends' produced a skit on the subject at our annual conference one year. But the scheme worked and I, too, could claim that my specialty was diarrhoea!

Chapter 7.

Some Difficult Dilemmas

Sad Story

S he was an attractive young Nepali wife adored by a fairly wealthy husband—and she had chronic renal failure. In those days there were no facilities for dialysis or kidney transplantation in Nepal, but I did what I could. Older physicians may recall the Bull-Borst regime which is all I had to offer. Actually a group of visiting German nephrologists had shaken their heads over the lack of dialysis equipment and had raised money to send several haemodialysis machines to the government hospital. These remained unopened in their crates for many years. After all there were not the trained personnel, laboratory resources or money to run them and renal failure is not a high priority in a country where infection and malnutrition are the main causes of death and disability. There is a lesson here for generous well-intentioned visitors; do a little wider research before you try to impose technology and change the health priorities of a struggling country.

To return to my patient; a hospital in Bombay was offering renal transplantation at the cost of 80,000 Indian rupees, then equivalent to about £5000 pounds, a staggering sum to most Nepalese especially as there would be the additional cost of flying the patient, relatives and kidney donor to Bombay and housing them there. However she was, as I say, a much loved wife and her husband had more means than most so he asked me what I thought.

This was a common and difficult dilemma for me. My instincts were all against it. Imagine me struggling day by day to make the best use of limited resources to help as many as possible, convinced that it was right to establish priorities and stick to them. To spend such a large sum on a procedure that might well not succeed was contrary to all my principles. On the other hand, I had to tell myself it was private money they were proposing to spend and it would not be available for other patients. If a man cares this much for his wife who is to stop him? My principles against their right to choose! Leaving aside the more philosophical aspects, I had worries about follow up even if the operation were to succeed. Graft rejection is a major concern and the necessary immunosuppressant drugs were expensive and not available in Nepal. There was no renal expertise and experience to deal with this in Nepal at that time and Bombay was more than a thousand miles away. I discussed it with them from all angles and concluded by advising them against going. Of course they went.

After a while they were back in Kathmandu and very happy indeed because the operation had gone well. There was a certain "I told you so" in the husband's relationships with me, though very gracious because that is the sort of people they are. Sadly, after a few months, graft rejection began to set in and gloom descended. I think there may have been another visit to Bombay but I'm not sure. Certainly she was back in my ward before many months had passed, so again I did what I could. We were clearly losing the battle. I asked if he wanted to take her back to Bombay, but his shoulders sagged; all his money had gone. She died and he was both bereft and impoverished. My instincts were right all along but it is sometimes a very painful thing to be right.

What is good medicine? Different countries have different philosophies. In the USA, it is possible to get any level of care, however expensive or technologically advanced, provided the patient can afford it or is adequately insured. As I wrote this in October 2013, the US government was in a state of shut down because one large political group would not approve the President's plan to make good health care available to the less well off. In the UK we have a health service that is funded by taxation and free at the point of delivery and this is a matter of national pride. However, taxation will never provide sufficient resources to keep up with all the technological advances and their accompanying high expense. Therefore the government has appointed a body to recommend what services may be provided under the National Health Service. The bottom line is that there must always be a rationing of services of some sort or other. Rationing is often thought to be a rude word in this context; let's call it 'priority setting'.

How much more necessary is some form of priority setting in a resource-poor country such as Nepal was and to some extent is still. At the time I am writing about, the government clinics were able to provide a limited range of free medicines and the annual supply of those usually ran out in a very few months. Other medicines would have to be bought at a 'Medical Hall', that is if there was one within a reachable distance and if the patient's family could afford it.

As I've already described, at Shanta Bhawan we were able to raise money for the treatment of the poor, some of it from gifts, some from our Robin Hood act with 'private' patients. But we still had to make hard choices and keep firm control of which services we were able to provide.

Dying Patients

I considered this dilemma more extensively in an article in the British Medical Journal which is reproduced as Appendix II.

There were cultural and religious aspects of death that I found hard to accommodate. It is generally felt that a Hindu should die in an auspicious place, ideally in a temple beside a river that eventually flows into the Ganges. The worst case scenario for some people was to die in a 'foreign' hospital and for the body to be touched by one of these people whose caste is so low they don't come into any known caste category. So if a patient seemed to be dying, the relatives would clamour to take him (or her) off to the 'ghat'. There, a special 'doctor', the *ghat vaidya*, would preside over the death. In the case of an old man with destroyed lungs and a failing heart, for example, I was reasonably happy to agree to his being taken away. It may not be fashionable any more, but I have always thought there was wisdom in the old saying "Thou shalt not kill–but do not strive officiously to keep alive". Many of my patients, however, were young people, perhaps with a severe septicaemia. It was not uncommon for them to go to the brink of death before finally responding to antibiotics, fluid replacement and other treatment They could go on to live normal lives. It was over patients like this that an unseemly tug of war could develop between relatives intent on taking the patient to the *ghat* and me, the doctor, trying to give the patient every chance of survival.

I recall an instance of this dilemma which occurred a year or two later. The patient was a young man employed by the national airline, then known as RNAC, the Royal Nepal Airlines Corporation. (The 'Royal' has now been dropped.) On that occasion, I won the tug of war and he recovered fully. There came a situation after he had returned to work that I was in Biratnagar, in the terai towards the west, needing a ticket for a flight to Kathmandu. I had been given a lift into Biratnagar from Dharan and needed to return there for the night. I was delighted to see that my former patient was manning the ticket desk in the small RNAC office, and I thought my business should go smoothly. He welcomed me with some joy and everyone who came into the office had to be told about his recovery and introduced to the 'Doctor Saheb'. This was gratifying, but had its down side; by the time these explanations and introductions had finished, my lift had gone and I was obliged to take a slow and tedious bus back to Dharan.

The Health Check—that makes you worse!

The wealthier Nepalese would go abroad for treatment or even for a health check-up. In 1982, I needed to accompany a Canadian colleague to a private hospital in Bangkok, Thailand. I will describe this in Chapter 12, but now I want to mention a Nepalese man that I met there. He had taken his wife for treatment and this seems to have been successful. However he thought it might be a good idea to have a full health check-up himself while he was there. He had a whole variety of scans and tests; from the point of view of a private, for profit institution that charges per item, the more tests the better! All was well except for a certain blood test, Alpha Fetoprotein or AFP, which was raised. AFP is a blood protein found in foetuses before birth, but there is not normally much of it in adult blood. Because of this, yet more tests were ordered, but were inconclusive. He was told that he might have a liver tumour, or perhaps cancer of his testis, but they could not be sure and he should come back again in six months' time to have the tests repeated. So a perfectly healthy man had his check-up, spent a large amount of money and went away terrified that he had a fatal tumour on the basis of a very unspecific test result.

I have always been a strong supporter of preventive medicine in all its forms, but this kind of health check-up is very largely a waste of funds and often without an evidence base. Even in the more developed countries there is currently a backlash against many screening programmes, including PSA for prostate cancer and even breast screening.

My working days were filled with questions like "What is appropriate?" And "Is this affordable?"

Chapter 8.

Sport and Recreation

This chapter is a rest from the various struggles to provide the medical services for needy Nepali folk. I have always needed some sport and exercise in my life and have been pleasantly surprised at the emphasis on this in recent years as part of a 'healthy lifestyle'. I would not want anyone to feel sorry for us; we had lots of fun!

Running

Not everyone feels the same, but running has always been a pleasure for me. In the early days in Nepal, it was possible simply to run out from our house onto paths between the rice fields and then even reach the foot of the mountains around the valley. There were pleasant paths by streams and rivers, over bridges, up and down small hills, past temples and small shrines and through the odd grassy field where no-one had got round to growing rice.

Unfortunately, the city spread outwards like wild fire and the pleasant paths became rough roads through houses, promising tracks became dead ends and at least some of the pleasure was taken out of it.

Running on the newly-built and almost deserted Ring Road used to be one of my special delights. For an account of the joys of running the ring road in 1981, please see Appendix IV. Alas, it is virtually impossible now.

Swimming

The climate was very encouraging for swimming activities, whether in hotel pools, lakes or rivers. We started the children at a very early age in a hotel pool, trying to fend off waiters offering drinks we could not afford. Also fending off the children, for whom a Coke was a great treat. But they took to swimming well and we had a lot of fun. There was also a public pool at Balaju, which was a treat, though a long way to go. I was amusing the children with 'flying angels', diving off the boards with them on my back, when an Indian said "Do more tricks with your baby". Jamie was not much more than that at the time. In fact, when we returned to UK for leave and went to swim in a public pool, he threw himself headlong into the deep end and the pool staff rushed up expecting to have to rescue him. He was only four and swam like a tadpole.

They later became national champions in their early teens! This was largely because there were very few Nepalese competitors in their age groups, but they won their races convincingly. [*Jamie says*: Yeah, thanks Dad….don't let it go to our heads!] I was also at the 'top level' at that time, but after the new national swimming association employed a Chinese swimming coach, Nepalese swimming made great steps forward and youngsters overtook me.

We all enjoyed camping holidays on the lake at Pokhara and would quite frequently swim across and back. On one occasion we were joined by the kids' former teacher, Ann Lycett and we were amused to see her swimming around a headland pursued by a swimming herd of buffalo!

Swimming rivers was a great challenge. They were so swift that you could expect to come to shore a long way downstream from where you started. World record time 400m swims were easily possible! Avoiding rocks was important and the eddies and rapids were quite dangerous. I remember swimming the Bhote Koshi with Mary on my back and wondering if I would make it safely to the other side. (Not that she couldn't have managed on her own!)

[*Jamie says*: In fact, Dad's own version of kayaking was also mainly river swimming, punctuated with occasional upside down canoeing.]

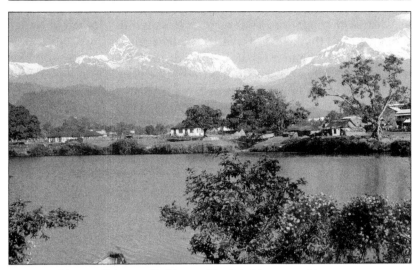

Phewa Tal near Pokhara. Photo: Maureen Newman

Basketball

Even when they were quite young, the children joined staff in playing basketball in a courtyard of Shanta Bhawan. Nepali doctors, including Buddha Basnyat and Kishore Pande would also play and were good with the children. Both kids later went to American-influenced schools and both got quite skilled. Mary even captained the Cambridge women's team against Oxford-the only time her mother and I shouted for the Light Blues!

The hospital entered tournaments run initially by the Jesuit-run, St Xavier's School (which Buddha and Kishore had both attended). However, in spite of one or two good players, we were not very good and usually got beaten early.

Tennis

I played quite a bit, but in the early days did not get nearly enough practice. I remember being invited to play in a 'top eight' tournament at a time when there were not many more players than that in the country. I greatly embarrassed myself on that occasion.

As with swimming, I soon got overtaken as tennis took off in Nepal, though I don't think I ever played as badly again.

Much later, I had a regular series of friendly matches with my friend Dick Harding. Dick was an American colleague in the mission who began as an internist but became a specialist in Community Health. At one point he had his mitral heart valve surgically replaced by a pig's valve. If he beat me, I would complain about being beaten by a pig! Over the years there were many other tennis partners and opponents; Korean, Russian, German, Irish, Canadian, Tibetan, Nepalese and others.

We were disappointed not to be able to interest the children in tennis at the time. Some 25 years later, Jamie said "Dad, teach me to play tennis" and now they are both playing with their own families.

Rugby

Rugby Union had very much been my winter sport at school and university. I stopped playing when I qualified; life was too busy and the consequences of an injury too great. There was no rugby in Nepal until a team from Armagnac in France came for a tour and wanted some opposition. The problems were formidable. A Hawaiian American tennis-playing friend made the arrangements and trained a team of expatriates most of whom had at least played the game before. I trained with them, but sadly injured my back before the two matches took place. It was necessary to use the football stadium in Kathmandu, but we had to clear a large number of stones off the pitch to make it more or less playable.

My part in the first match was to run the line with a sponge and some emergency kit, and I think I spent more time on the pitch than many of our players! The French proved highly competitive and pushed the Laws to their limit and beyond. We were quite a puny opposition, but they showed no mercy.

In the second match, I was asked to take a microphone and explain to the crowd in Nepali what was going on. This was very necessary as rugby had never been played in Nepal before. The problem was to find a suitable vocabulary with which to describe it. "Scrum *bhayo*" seemed a bit feeble! In spite of complete ignorance of the Laws, the audience had a great time, cheering lustily whenever a player disappeared under a horde of tacklers, or got knocked off his feet in open play. Many bottles of the local produce of Armagnac were generously distributed after the match.

Trekking

One activity which did not go down well with the children in their early years was trekking. Their attitude was "Why are we doing this?" Surrounded by fabulous mountain scenery, camping in idyllic spots beside streams and rivers, they were singularly unimpressed.

All this changed when they went to boarding school in the Indian Himalaya. Not only did they need to climb 500 feet from their dormitories to the school, but also the main school leisure activity was hiking. Doing it with their friends, very often with no staff supervision, they wandered all over the hills and found themselves really enthusiastic about an activity they had previously despised!

On their school holidays, trekking with parents or with friends in Nepal became a much-loved activity. They would come home at the beginning of the monsoon period for the long school holiday and we would try to do a 'beat the monsoon' hike. It rarely worked! We would usually come home soaked and with many leech bites. On one occasion, Mary counted up to 100 leeches on her before she gave up counting!

School Holiday Activities

At other seasons, we would do different and longer treks. I was expected to have at least one adventure lined up for them when they came back from school. One was particularly successful, but complicated. I had quite a good relation with the Mountain Travel organisation, who also ran the Tiger Tops jungle lodges. On one previous occasion, we had gone there for me to do some medical work with their staff and the family to enjoy elephant rides, the one-horned rhinoceros and tigers. (To be truthful, I got my chance as well!) This time I arranged that we would visit the Tharu Village site, not so much for the wild life as for the interesting character of the Tharu people. They have lived in the forested Terai for generations in spite of the virulent malaria which decimated other visitors to the forest. This particular year, I put on a three-part adventure; we travelled down to the Terai by raft on the white water Trisuli and Narayani rivers, stayed a few days in the Tharu village and then took a bus to Hetauda where we were met by Saila and his friends to trek our way back into the Kathmandu Valley.

As a precursor of this adventure, the children got back from school not knowing that the following day they would be running the full 17 mile circuit of the Ring Road on a charity run to raise money for Patan Hospital.

Running

I was really proud of both of them on that run. I think Mary finished as the second female and I can't just remember if she was 14 or 15. Jamie, two years younger, completely inexperienced but fresh from his frequent exertions up and down the hills at school, set off at a tremendous pace and left me well behind. I feared he would not manage to finish the course and, indeed, I passed him after a few miles. However, he completed the entire course which was a considerable achievement at that age. [*Jamie adds:*–and finished ahead of his sister!!!! – phew needed to get that in.] Angela chose the rescue Land Rover! She also had to minister to three exhausted relatives when we got home and collapsed, all three, on the double bed.

Rafting

Next day it was off on a bus to the place where we were to enter the Trisuli River. Krishna, our raft captain gave us safety equipment and a quick guide to rafting, including instructions as to what to do if you fell in the water. (Go downstream feet first until you reach a quiet stretch and can be rescued!)

The river was quite lively, with frequent rapids which we were taught to negotiate and some more placid gentle stretches surrounded by wonderful scenery. We noticed a few isolated, sandy beaches and were delighted to find that we were to camp on one of them. However three of us, still feeling our aching limbs from the run the day before, groaned a bit when Krishna suggested a walk to a village, some way off. Still, we managed it somehow and returned for an evening meal under the stars and a peaceful night.

Next day there were more rapids on the Trisuli before we came to the Narayani River. This is a mighty tributary of the Ganges and, as the Kali Gandaki in its upper reaches, passes through the deepest gorge on earth between the Annapurna range and Mount Dhaulagiri. We were treated to a gentler, wider run down through the Siwalik Hills to the Chitwan Valley and the Tharu Village camp. The Village was a quiet cultural interlude in which we saw something of the life of the Tharu, their artwork and especially their dancing.

And trekking

Then it was off by bus through the flat Terai to Hetauda, where, with some difficulty, we met up with Saila and two other porters who had brought tents and camping equipment by bus from Kathmandu. Before any real roads were built in Nepal, the main route to Kathmandu from the Indian border led through Hetauda and Bhimpedi and we wanted to follow this historical route. The Ranas and the royal family, the Shahs, used to import from India Rolls Royces and other vehicles, which they ran on the few roads in the Kathmandu Valley. To do this, of course, the vehicles had to be stripped down to smaller parts and then carried by teams of porters up this very path. At the time we walked it, the route was used to bring buffalo into the Kathmandu Valley to be offered as sacrifices to the goddess Kali at the great *Dasain* festival. Buffalo were not designed to walk for days on stony paths and their feet and hooves were liable to damage, so their drovers fashioned boots of straw for their protection. The path was littered in places by discarded buffalo boots.

Though in the middle of winter, the weather in the lowlands was quite hot and the cold water at a hilltop place called Chisapani was very welcome. (*Chisapani* means cold water and *Tatopani* means hot water, or hot springs.)

We had a memorable, if unconventional, Christmas Day lunch by a large reservoir at Khulkhani. It featured specially hoarded spam, if I remember rightly. Then we proceeded up and over the last range into the Kathmandu Valley and home. An eventful Christmas holiday, and I think the children may think this kind of thing compensated for any deprivation they may have felt from being brought up in the Himalaya.

Amateur Dramatics

In those early days, there was no live entertainment, no TV and very few cinemas. Nepalis were good at putting on 'cultural programmes' consisting of songs, dances and some skits, but there were no plays except those put on by the Himalayan Amateurs, (HAMS). HAMS had both Nepalese and expatriate members, but probably the expats were more numerous. When we managed to find a bit of leisure time after the first few years, Angela and I took part in a few productions. Angela did a very good Wicked Witch of the West in "The Wizard of Oz". [*Mary says:* No kidding, the local kids were scared of her for years afterwards!] We both enjoyed taking part in "My Three Angels" a play about prisoners on Devil's Island and we learnt the long parts involved to play Norman and Ethel in "On Golden Pond". [Mary says: Dad still wears what we call his "Norman hat" to keep the sun off his head. He's probably just about now getting to the kind of age where it's appropriate to wear it.] This play was enjoyable, but the advent of video machines and the recording of Henry Fonda and Kathleen Hepburn in the film while we were in rehearsal meant that the audience was smaller than we would have liked. HAMS found itself with competition for the first time.

I enjoyed singing in Gilbert and Sullivan's "The Pirates of Penzance". [*Mary says:* Singing?!] For some reason, my singing has always been a source of amusement. I was a pirate in the first half and a policeman in the second. Nepalese friends came to see it and found it hilarious and colourful, but probably understood only a small fraction of what was going on. There was an event during rehearsals that had both a tragic and a comic side. An American friend was also in the police chorus. On the way to rehearsal one filthy, wet night, he stopped his car at a traffic light and a cycle rickshaw crashed into the back of it. Onto the road spilled a man carrying a child in his arms and unfortunately the child suffered a severe head injury. My friend put both of them into his car and drove them to the government hospital, where he was promptly arrested. This was standard; the driver was always assumed to be at fault. Sadly, the child died and my friend remained in custody. He was quite friendly with his guards, though, and it was agreed that he should be allowed to take part in the performances under police guard. So we had the extraordinary sight of an American on stage dressed in British bobby uniform, watched from the wings by his uncomprehending Nepalese guard in his uniform of khaki shorts and shirt! I'm glad to say that, after some weeks, he was released.

My tennis-playing American Friend, Dr Dick Harding, sang the part of Rafe Rackstraw in "HMS Pinafore". I couldn't help being amused as the chorus sang to him "For he is an Englishman!"

Angela wants to mention the AWON library, an excellent collection of books left behind by ex-patriates. We all took out a life membership but found when we returned in 2000 that it had expired!

Visitors

One advantage of living in a country with a romantic image is that interesting people come to stay with you! Of course there were memorable visits from various family and friends as well as mission folk from other countries, but I want to mention a few rather high-profile medical folk that I might well have not met otherwise.

Moran Campbell was a renowned respiratory physician who, having done important research at the Hammersmith Hospital in London moved to Canada as Professor of Medicine at the innovative Medical School at McMaster University in Ontario. Moran and his wife, Diana, came and stayed with us. We didn't keep alcohol in the house, partly out of financial necessity and partly because the Nepali church was very much against it. But an evening gin and tonic was an essential for Moran and Diana, so he went to the bazaar and found some gin (probably from India) and a lemon drink that made a suitable mixer. Moran was also keen to go on a trek and found out rather late in the day that he needed a trekking permit and for this he needed a passport photo, which he didn't have. I guess one tall white man looks much the same as another, so I gave him a photo of me and it was never questioned!

A giant of a figure in the history of tuberculosis was Sir John Crofton. He was Professor of Respiratory Diseases at Edinburgh University, President of the Royal College of Physicians of Edinburgh and author of a major book on respiratory disease. His group in Edinburgh was responsible for recognizing that treatment with streptomycin alone leads to drug resistance and failure and for the development of treatment with three drugs to prevent relapse and resistance. After his retirement, he travelled to many countries advising on TB, including Nepal. He sometimes stayed with us and came on ward rounds with me at Shanta Bhawan giving a lot of valuable help and advice. In spite of arthritis in his hips, he was apparently happy to be transported around Kathmandu on the back of my motor cycle. These things are supposed to be secret, but I am fairly certain that it was he who nominated me for the Fellowship of the Royal College of Physicians (of London, not Edinburgh). Perhaps this arose out of relief at surviving my motor bike and the Kathmandu traffic!

Stephen Lock was Editor of the British Medical Journal from 1975 to 1991. He also came to visit us with some medical friends connected with the Journal and doubtless this had something to do with my getting some articles published in the 70s and 80s.

One of Stephen's friends was Alex Paton, whom I got to know quite well and who later entertained me in his home near Birmingham. I think he was the original 'Minerva'. Minerva, the Roman goddess of wisdom, medicine and a variety of other things, has contributed an anonymous back page to the BMJ for many years. Only recently did I discover that Alec was a medical student at St Thomas's Hospital in London at the end of the Second World War and volunteered with others to help with the horrendous medical and humanitarian crisis that followed the discovery of appalling conditions left by the Nazis at the Belsen prison camp. (Paton, 1981)

Chapter 9.

Rock and Wait (The kid's perspective). By Jamie

Rocking and Waiting

I don't know personally, but I'm told that the life of a rock and roll star is all about Rock and Wait; wild excitement on stage juxtaposed with long periods in airport lounges, tour buses and a lot of hanging around before the next gig. I can relate to the Rock and Wait theme growing up in Kathmandu with a raft of amazing experiences including – er–rafting obviously, kayaking, trekking, riding on the roof rack of buses through Himalayas, amazing places, friends and interesting people.

The views, the colourful culture, adventure, the wildlife (and only slightly domesticated animals like our dog Gyp), and the possibilities for mischief, diversion and general teenage kicks were amazing. There was the freedom to ride a motorbike on the roads aged 14, options for all kinds of epic journeys, a variety of entertainment courtesy of the missionary and international communities and of course amazing hospitality from Nepali people.

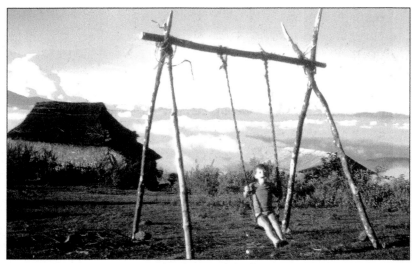

Jamie on a 'Ping'

And then there was waiting. Waiting for electricity, so that I could play with a new toy. Waiting for months for chums to return from their furlough in their native Australia, New Zealand, or U.S. Sometimes waiting nearly all day for a working bus with a working driver or most elusively a passable road. All that possibility made the waiting so difficult. I could wait for trips to the UK for TV, cinema and the English version of youth activities. But even as an adult returning to Kathmandu in my 30's I couldn't control myself sitting on the plane on the tarmac at Tribhuwan Airport waiting for the stairs to be driven up to the aircraft, and tried to make a break for it. The stewardess gave me a good ticking off for trying to leg it into Nepal before the 'fasten seat belts' sign was turned off.

Nepal didn't have a monopoly on boring, far from it. Going from church to church in the UK hearing my parents do the same spiel about "living in Nepal" would definitely progress through the rounds of "Britain's got Boring" if the judges heard it as many times as I did. It was more that Nepal offered the tantalising prospect of adventure and exhilaration round the corner, while we spent the day queuing for a bottle of gas for cooking or waited for Mum to finish gassing with missionaries as part of her job with the induction programme – or possibly just because that's what she likes to do.

And if waiting the time it takes to drive up the truck with the aeroplane steps is bad, it's a mere couple of minutes compared to Nepali church services where Pastor Robert Karthak easily managed prayers of 37 minutes and 18 seconds (my friend Sniffs and I timed him one Christmas Day), and sermons of up to 110 minutes. To my shame, my Nepali language extends to useful expressions for playing games with kids in the street, for shopping, hiking, or drinking and a few useful phrases for keeping out of trouble with authorities. Under pressure I could manage "I'm very sorry officer" (a particular favourite of my grandfather) and once topped it with the extremely audacious and bizarrely successful; "Oh no! I'm not riding this motorbike without a helmet or a licence; I'm just out taking it somewhere I can learn to ride properly".

But my ineptitude with Nepali meant I didn't understand anything at all with spiritual or religious vocabulary. So I missed the subtleties. In fact I missed Pastor Robert's point, theme, and entire topic even, and all the while completely failed to sit comfortably on the ground. Even in primary school I lacked the flexibility or balance to manage a proper crossed-legs sit. Flopping in a less formal, organised way was also problematic though. There are ways of causing offence with your feet, legs, "dirty", left hand, and (where caste is taken seriously) just touching someone who is high caste. Nepali politeness means that it may not even be mentioned, but it causes awkwardness nonetheless. I remember being sprawled out on a tea shop veranda one lunchtime after a hard morning trekking uphill; completely oblivious to the fact that I was effectively pinning the owner's daughter in the corner as it would have been embarrassing for her to step over me.

So I never mastered sitting cross legged despite this coming naturally to every Nepali aged more than a few months old. I would have loved to have been cool like the Nepali people and hippies and think that *sukals* (straw mats), carpets or floors made of fired clay and cow dung are all comfortable, appealing places to sit in a tea shop, guesthouse or Nepali church –but no. I'm acculturated in other ways, and to me a squat toilet is a very welcome sight in any corner of the globe, but I just can't sit cross legged on the floor.

My manners must have been appalling. I've griped, whined and generally been a spoiled western brat about fleas in the *sukal* biting me while our Nepali hosts were lavishing a lot more on us than they could afford to spend. I've attended weddings and been far more interested in stray dogs and barely noticed the bride and groom. What's more, my limited attention span and floor-sitting challenges meant that going to someone's house for dinner became the ultimate ordeal of waiting. In fact, I doubt they would admit it, but I think it was the ultimate ordeal of waiting for the rest of my family; in Nepal the format of a dinner invitation is that you arrive hours before anyone even starts on the meal [*Dad says:* The chicken was probably still running about outside!] Many hours later, food is eventually produced. You tuck in, and literally put your plate down and nip off home straight away.

Offering huge amounts of food is polite in Nepal and pretty much de rigueur. You can try refusing second helpings, but you are unlikely to be taken seriously. You can put your hands over your plate only to find your host pouring rice between your fingers. Nothing you can do will stop the friendliest, smiling, insanely-hard-to-refuse and certainly not-taking-"no"- for -an -answer host from feeding you.

Of course I didn't manage to disgrace myself in the unique way Dad managed on one occasion. He ended up having an asthma attack at a party from overeating and needed the 15 year old stick thin me weighing practically nothing to ride him home on his motorbike while he wheezed, choked and tried not to pass out. I can't say that evening was boring.

In Mussoorie too

School similarly felt mundane with the Himalaya as a playground. Mary and I went to secondary school in India, but still in the Himalayan foothills. This was considered a safe place for boys and we were afforded a remarkable amount of freedom. Sure, buses plunged over huge drops where landslides eroded the roads, drugs were freely available, my grasp of Hindi is even worse than my Nepali and I have no sense of direction whatsoever, but the school allowed me to disappear for the weekend with two equally linguistically and navigationally challenged buddies. In spite of everything, we managed to get back to school for classes on the following Monday. [*Mum says:* See footnote in chapter 3–lots of people were praying!] Generally we did actually go to our logged destination, but these were fairly outrageous in themselves and involved route marching through the night, hopping trucks and ascending peaks. Groups with girls needed chaperones, but from the age of 12 boys could roam virtually anywhere there wasn't a big city – which leaves a whole lot of India. Our freedom was slightly restricted after my sister's hiking party returned three days late from an attempt to cross a high pass over the source of the Ganges with frostbitten chaperones. So when my intrepid chums and I attempted it, the school insisted we took a guide (who incidentally turned out to be a drug fiend). Sadly we had to turn back when waist high snow even on lower reaches made our progress impossible.

One treat the school had was a surprise holiday to celebrate the end of the monsoon, by which time everyone is feeling cooped up and ready to get themselves outdoors and do something. I'm yet to experience waking up on a damp Monday morning with the prospect of a dismal week, to half-heartedly check a lottery ticket from Saturday and find that... Well obviously that hasn't happened to me yet, but I do have a sort of idea of the kind of emotion involved courtesy of Woodstock School's "fair weather holiday". After four and a half months of monsoon, the Head Teacher would try to ascertain that on that particular day the rain had finally stopped. Plans were usually disguised for as long as possible. Sometimes we would sit all the way through assembly until the glorious bombshell was dropped; that, for today, school is cancelled through lack of interest. To a schoolboy, obviously this is the best thing that could ever happen. One minute we were dreading double maths, the incomplete homework, the forgotten PE kit; the next minute we were celebrating and discovering the hidden reserves of *joie de vivre* you can have on a day jumping in the back of a passing truck and stowing away. Then hiking to a river for a swim or to float over rapids in a car inner tube, and inevitably find somewhere to consume *barfi, jalebi, kulfi, gulab jamun* and other Indian treats. Of course it usually rained on the fair weather holiday, but it didn't matter because we were having fun.

Back in Nepal there were similar occasions when all the signs predicted a grim time ahead, but somehow everything I expected was utterly wrong, and I got something entirely different from what I had envisioned.

Anandaban

I could start talking about how on the face of it, the idea of trekking with mission doctors who on a daily basis seemed overwrought and cantankerous didn't appeal much. Once trekking somehow the aspect morphed into frat –boy life and soul of the party and outstandingly good entertainment value. But I wanted to mention perhaps the most remarkable example of when I expected the worst, but ended up really enjoying myself; visiting the leprosy hospital, Anandaban. *Anandaban* translates as "forest of joy", and although it sounds like a euphemism or a bit twee – it actually felt like a holiday resort. If the Star Ship Enterprise hologram suite is programmed properly you would say "computer–forest of joy!"–and you should get something very similar to Anandaban.

I might struggle to sell a leprosy hospital as a weekend getaway, but it was surprisingly luxurious, starting with very reasonable transfers. A typical journey in and around Kathmandu could involve a trolley bus heaving full of people, goats, chickens, and inevitably some vomit. An ordinary Nepali bus is similarly crowded with a wider variety of animals and more vomit. Bus journeys take forever with much waiting. You would circle Ratna Park a few times being ushered on to random buses by someone with a tenuous relationship with the bus company. Eventually the real driver would show up, but need *dal bhat*, tea and cigarettes before doing anything. Finally the ignition would be tried and nothing would happen. Once jump started, the herd of goats on board would be swapped for a different herd, and once this crucial change had been accomplished the bus would creep slowly towards our destination.

Anandaban by contrast is just a short hop from Patan Hospital of about an hour or so and all of the first four or five minutes of the drive as I remember it is on a tarmacked road. The rutted road didn't matter too much, because this time we were travelling first class in a *"gari"* (usually a Land Rover), still obviously somewhat like a Japanese train after the packers have finished stuffing in all of Tokyo's morning commuters, but a limousine in contrast to our usual ride.

The accommodation (and I think to be fair we were honoured guests) was clean, comfortable and charming on the edge of the wood and a short walk from the hospital. The forest had walks that even my sister and I enjoyed and distracted us from sulking. There were sports facilities for table tennis, volleyball and football and lots of cheery staff and patients to play with. I don't know a lot about leprosy, but used to be moderately horrified by amputees begging on Kathmandu's main drag, New Road. Here, people seemed optimistic, contented and happy. They also demonstrated some mean ping pong skills. Every time we went there, I would rethink about how I viewed "sick" and "well".

In contrast to Anandaban's tranquillity I had a hair-raising encounter with a health care connection years later when I visited Nepal during the period when Maoists in the hills engaged in kidnapping and extortion. I had borrowed a motorbike and was on a long ride when I was stopped by a *bandh* style barrier across the road and some guys who styled their look on Che Guevara. "We want your blood!" one fellow shouted at me in English. Fortunately this was a mistranslation and he explained in Nepali using a few visual clues that he wanted me to give a financial donation ostensibly to the blood bank. I've never been so happy to hand over cash.

Something for everyone?

Even in the 00's Nepali youth were having 70's style "happenings" which I sampled and judged to be "groovy". But if this isn't your bag (man) I'd encourage you to go and float an inner tube or a kayak down a river, or paddle a plastic bath across a paddy field, have "kite fights" with broken glass on the string so you "cut down" your opponents kite for the local children to chase after. Have paint chucked over you in the Holi celebration or check out the guys going round singing at Tihar (Diwali). (A bit like carollers, but a different month and singing *"Do-si-le"* and *"Bhailo"* instead of "We Three Kings".) Smell the incense and flowers in a Hindu puja. Take a flight where you are completely convinced the plane is about to land in the car park; oh no that's actually the runway. Be amazed at how the bus driver navigates a tiny winding, collapsing road at great speed with endless drops on both sides. There may be some waiting involved, but Nepal has a lot to offer.

As I write, Nepal is in the middle of even more difficult times. In the aftermath of the February 2015 earthquake, Everest has only just opened again—and tourism has slowed to a trickle. But Nepal has unique thrills and experiences. The far out generation who came seeking far out experiences when I was there growing up found the drugs, mysticism and alternate life in this place they had imagined when they were listening to Jimi Hendrix. More recently, the extreme sports enthusiasts , adventure seekers, trekkers and climbers find plenty that is "rad" and "knarly", but you don't have to subscribe to a particular lifestyle to find Nepal enchanting and captivating. My family did – keep reading!

Chapter 10.

Mountain Sickness; because it's there!

Famously, when asked why he wanted to climb Mount Everest, George Mallory replied "Because it's there"! I suppose that's the answer to why I studied acute mountain sickness and high altitude physiology. There I was, at Shanta Bhawan, a hospital at the relatively modest altitude of 4,200 feet or so, but the hospital to which foreigners especially were evacuated by helicopter when problems arose on a trek in the Himalaya or on an expedition to climb one of the massive peaks.

I had barely heard of acute mountain sickness! There was little written about it in 1969 when I first went to Nepal, though names like *'puna'* and *'soroche'* had been used in the Andes for centuries. Chinese sources referred to the 'Headache Mountains' of Tibet and the Karakorum. Nepalese simply refer to being *'lekh lageko'*, affected by the mountains.

T H Ravenhill, a mine doctor in Peru, in a paper in 1913, described *'Puna'* as having a 'normal type' in which headache, nausea, vomiting, chest discomfort and dizziness predominated, a 'Cardiac Type' with much breathlessness, and a 'Nervous Type' which had neurological symptoms. The 'Cardiac Type' proved to be more a problem of the lungs than the heart.

In 1970, a South Korean mountaineer was brought down by heli-copter from the approaches to Mount Lhotse, a near neighbour of Everest. From the airport he was brought to Shanta Bhawan. He was deeply unconscious and remained so for three weeks, after which he gradually improved. For a further period he was severely disorien-tated, at one point appearing to mistake the whitewashed walls of the hospital for the ice cliffs of Lhotse! I found out later that he recov-ered fully back in Korea. This was my first experience of what is now generally called High Altitude Cerebral Oedema, which equates with Ravenhill's 'Nervous Type' and which I prefer to call Cerebral Acute Mountain Sickness. (I think I lost the battle over the terminology!)

His case contrasts with that of a climber brought down from Everest Base Camp by Peter Steele who was doctor to the ill-fated International Expedition of 1971. (Steele 1972). This patient was severely breathless during the previous day and night, but, as the heli-copter brought him to lower altitudes, he removed his oxygen mask and was virtually normal by the time he arrived at the hospital. Not so, his doctor! Peter had stumbled while carrying an oxygen cylinder across the Khumbhu Glacier at Base Camp and developed severe pain in his chest! I diagnosed a rupture of the junction between a rib and the cartilage that joins it to the breastbone; painful, but self-healing in time.

This second patient had High Altitude Pulmonary Oedema, Ravenhill's 'Cardiac Type' and my Pulmonary Acute Mountain Sickness.

The third form is officially just known as Acute Mountain Sickness, Ravenhill's 'Normal Type'. I prefer to call it 'Benign Acute Mountain Sickness' as it is not fatal in itself, though it may lead to one or both of the more severe forms if it is not managed correctly. The proper management is for the patient to climb no higher until recovered and to descend if there is any evidence of deterioration.

Patients kept coming from high altitude during the trekking and mountaineering seasons and sadly seven of them died. Others died in the Himalaya and were buried under a pile of stones. Dr Walter Bond did meticulous autopsies on those that died in the hospital and these formed a basis for my thesis on the subject some 11 years after my first examination of the unconscious Korean.

It became obvious that Germans and Japanese formed a dispro-portionate number of the victims. Of the 57 that I was able to study (including the fatal cases) 22 were German or Austrian and seven Japanese. I speculated that this might reflect the determination of these races to press upward at all costs, even when disabled by mountain sickness. There was only one Sherpa and he was taken ill very high on Everest. The only other Nepalese was a lady who had been on a pilgrimage to the high Gosainkund lakes north of Kathmandu.

Himalayan Rescue Association

Some of us had a concern over the number of people who were going into the mountains without any real understanding of the dangers. I was shocked to find several Alpine guides among the victims of mountain sickness. They simply had not realised that the Himalaya more or less begins at the altitude of the highest peaks in the Alps. In the interests of what would nowadays be known as 'awareness-raising', we founded the Himalayan Rescue Association. http://www.himalayanrescue.org

The main initiative came from John Skow, who had been a Peace Corps Volunteer from the USA. After various discussions, HRA was formed and consisted of John Skow, Tek Chandra Pokharel, a travel and tours operator, Robert Reiffel, the local manager of Air France, Mike Cheney and Dawa Norbu Sherpa of Mountain Travel with me as Medical Adviser. It was not feasible for us to go rushing into the high Himalaya to rescue climbers or mountaineers in distress in the way that local rescue groups do in Europe. Our first task was to develop a leaflet for high altitude tourists, trekkers and climbers explaining the dangers of altitude and advising simple but necessary precautions; plan carefully, do not climb too much each day, be prepared to stay where you are if you get sick, or descend if it is bad or getting worse. We defined a sensible rate of ascent; above 3000m sleep no higher than 300-400m above the previous night's altitude and take 'rest days' at about 3000m and 4000m on which you sleep no higher than you did the night before. We had hoped that this leaflet could be distributed by the government with trekking permits, but the authorities did not like the idea of telling prospective tourists that there might be danger and so putting them off.

The next step was to found an HRA Aid Post at Pheriche at 4400m on the Everest trekking route. This was manned by expatriate volunteers and opened in a yak hut in 1974. A permanent building was completed in 1975. A further Aid Post was opened on the Manang trekking route.

A transient expertise

Because 'it' was there, and I was there, I became known as an expert in mountain sickness. In 1975, I published a paper on 'A Cerebral Form of High Altitude Illness' in the Lancet with Dr Charlie Houston with whom I had been corresponding. It contained descriptions of several of my cases from Shanta Bhawan and some autopsy results. It was probably the first descriptive paper on the subject since Ravenhill's. Also in 1975, Charlie invited me to a conference on Mountain Medicine in the Yosemite National Park in California in the dead of winter. I was due some leave, but mission doctors do not have enough in the bank to buy air tickets to the USA. However the Mountain Travel company in Nepal was also the GSA for Pan American Airlines in Nepal and Jim Edwards, the Chairman, kindly provided exactly what I needed, a round the world air ticket.

The Yosemite conference was the first of several that I was able to attend in North America, but was memorable in many ways. The scenic grandeur of the great rock faces, El Capitan and Half Dome and others, the new friendships with a number of people who were interested in high altitude medicine and physiology and also meeting with a historic character, Noel Odell, who was a guest of honour.

Noel was a geologist at Cambridge and elsewhere, but he was also a member of the 1924 British Everest expedition from the North. This is well known for the loss of George Mallory and Andrew (Sandy) Irvine and the ongoing uncertainty whether they reached the summit or not. Odell's feat was remarkable; he was the last person to see them alive and spent two weeks above 23,000ft without extra oxygen. Twice he climbed to 26 800ft during that time. It is distinctly possible in retrospect to believe that the climb would have been successful if he had been partnered with Mallory instead of the younger and less experienced Irvine. I calculate that he was 85 at the time that I met him and he died aged 97.

To Everest Base Camp in a Great Man's Boots

Possibly because of my experience with mountain sickness, I was invited to go as Medical Officer on a trek run by Cook's Tours to the Solu Khumbu area and the Everest Base Camp in 1972. This was a great treat as all expenses were paid and I was able to make one of the great treks without any financial cost and whilst it was still virtually unspoiled. (I would not want to do it today!)

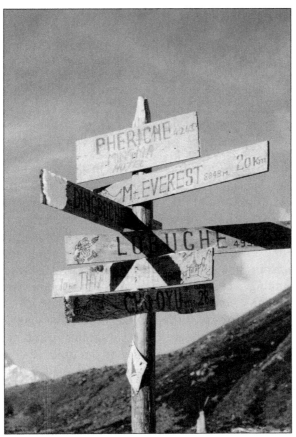

Signpost at Pheriche. Photo: Dr Gerry Hankins

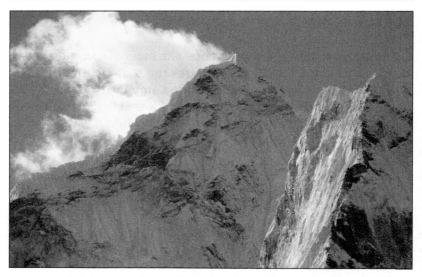

Clouds wreathing Mt Nuptse. Photo : Dr Gerry Hankins

It was quite a luxurious trek and I was first introduced to the way Nepali guides, Sherpas and porters take an almost feudal care of their charges. Hot drinks are always waiting at stopping places, lunch is always ready at a pre-defined and usually delightful spot, tents have been erected at the night's camp site, an excellent evening meal is served around a fire and , in the morning, there is 'bed tea' and hot water for washing and shaving. Needless to say, trekkers did not need to carry anything except a small day pack. (The doctor was an exception—I had to carry emergency kit.)

I first met the group at the Shanker Hotel and was a little concerned when one lady appeared to be breathless climbing the steps to the hotel door. However, she did manage quite well in the end, though others didn't. I was introduced as an 'expert' in mountain sickness and one-by-one over the next few days, the members sidled up to me and expressed their anxieties about this threat. While we were still at very low altitude, one young man came to me complaining of breathlessness at night and was sure he had pulmonary oedema. It transpired that he and his tent mate had closed up their tent so tightly that their expired air could not escape and they were feeling the effects of re-breathing carbon dioxide.

Unlike the others, who were superbly well-equipped, I had only an old and battered pair of boots that I hoped would survive the trek. They didn't! Approaching Namche Bazaar, the sole of one boot came very loose and dropped off. None of the local Sherpas seemed to have any ability to repair boots, so I took a side trip to the hospital that Sir Edmund Hillary had built for the Sherpas at Khunde, thinking there might be some expertise there. None at all as it turned out, but to my delight Ed himself was there; the first time I had met him. As we sat on a veranda, he heard of my boot problem and said "No worries, you can have a pair of mine–they're a bit too small anyway." Apparently they were only size 13! Thus it was that I went to Everest Base Camp in Ed Hillary's boots and several pairs of socks!

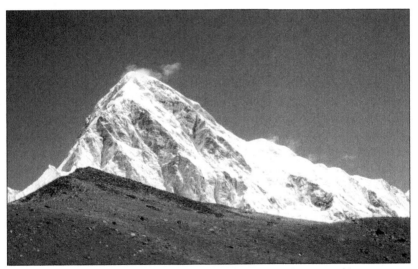

The 'Black Rock' and Mt Pumori. Photo: Dr Gerry Hankins

As we got within a day's trek of Everest, I got busier caring for the trekkers. Mostly, it was just tiredness, and one person had to be left to recover with a Sherpa at the penultimate camp at Lobuche. One youngish lady, who had been going strongly all the time and was eager to get to the Base Camp, suddenly lost the sight in one eye. This was beyond my experience, though a few other cases were later described elsewhere and it became part of the spectrum of acute high altitude illnesses. I did not dare take a chance and I accompanied her back down to the camp below, which was at Pheriche. There I am glad to say that she recovered her sight fully and, though desperately disappointed, she agreed that I had made the correct decision. The later cases also turned out to be fully reversible as far as I know.

However, I then had to walk the double stage, Pheriche to Lobuche and Lobuche to the Base Camp, where I caught up with the main party. One of them had apparently collapsed into his tent on arrival and didn't emerge until the next morning, when he stretched and, faced by the magnificent circle of peaks, enquired "Which is Everest?" Then he retreated back into the tent.

Having ascertained that all was well, I could not resist climbing to the superb viewpoint of Kala Patthar, the 'Black Rock' from which Charlie Houston and his father, with Bill Tillman the British Explorer had, in 1950, looked up across the Khumbu Glacier and the Western Cwm to the South Col. As the world knows, this proved a feasible route, and Hillary and Tensing completed it in 1953 in time for our Queen's coronation.

My trek on that long day was still not over. I needed to return to the lady that we had left at Lobuche and ensure that she was recovering, as indeed she was. It was getting dark as I walked alone down the trail. Looking up, I saw a huge shape towering over me, white with a conical head and dark sturdy legs. I could feel the adrenaline hit me in the back of my neck. The Yeti! However a second look showed that it was merely a snow covered rock, with a bare area in the centre, which my tired mind and body had interpreted as an animal shape. Reaching Lobuche, I collapsed into my tent and enjoyed a meal and my sleeping bag.

Passing on the knowledge

Various trekking doctors and others came to me for advice about mountain sickness. I have always been delighted when the 'disciple' has overtaken and exceeded the 'master's achievements and this was the case with at least two of these in the mountain medicine arena.

Dr Peter Hackett is an American who came to Nepal with a trekking group in 1974 and knew next to nothing about mountain sickness. I was able to meet with him and later corresponded. We met on his subsequent visits to Nepal and he took over the position of Medical

Director to the HRA and did stints as the volunteer doctor at Pheriche. He did some very good epidemiological research on mountain sickness in the Khumbhu region, interviewing and studying the trekkers as they passed through Pheriche. In perhaps his peak achievement, he climbed to the summit of Everest on the 24th October 1981. He was part of the American Medical Research Expedition to Mount Everest, reaching the summit alone and falling on the descent in a way that could have been fatal. Fortunately, his boot caught on a rock and, though suspended upside down he managed to recover using a fixed rope left by another expedition. (West, 1982)

He had many more achievements and appointments in the fields of mountain and wilderness medicine.

Dr Buddha Basnyat, in contrast, is Nepalese. As I have described, he came to me at Shanta Bhawan Hospital for his internship in medicine after graduating from the University of Patiala in the Punjab. With his cheerful good nature and interest in all things medical, he became a reliable colleague and close friend. [*Mary says: ...and favourite basketball player when we were kids.*] He eventually took over two of my 'mantles'; the first as head of physiology at the medical school and secondly as the Nepal authority in mountain medicine. Starting with the patients that we saw together, he developed an interest in altitude research and published important papers. He was one of the first to take an interest in the welfare of porters on trekking parties and expeditions. These form a group ignored by most people, but Buddha championed their interests. He gained such a name internationally that he was elected President of the International Society of Mountain Medicine (ISMM). He also, in turn, became Medical Director of HRA.

I claim no credit for the fine achievements of these two men, but I am very glad to have played a small part in the development of their interests.

Return to the Khumbhu

I got an invitation from the World Bank to go on an all-expenses-paid trip to the Everest region. The object was to write a report on the medical facilities available in the area as part of the World

Bank- funded project to create the Mount Everest National Park. This was too good to be missed!

I was able to secure the services of Saila as my porter and cook (Saila, with his father, appears in the TB tales.) Instead of walking in to the Khumbu, as I had with the Cook's Tour, we flew into the airfield at Lukla, lying at about 9,000ft. The grass runway is at a 30° angle. Landing is, of course, uphill and, on take-off, planes fly off the edge of a cliff and zoom *downwards* as they gain the speed to climb over the ridge on the other side of the valley. Scattered wrecks of aircraft did little to instil confidence.

However it was a pleasure to be safe and sound and back in the high mountains again. We camped by streams and visited various facilities, including the Khunde Hospital and the HRA Aid Post at Pheriche. As it happened, Peter Hackett was doing a stint there and gave me a full account of activities. I wanted a photograph illustrating how mountain sickness victims were evacuated with oxygen cylinders on the backs of yaks. There were no real victims, so I had to ride the yak. Now the yak is a tetchy sort of creature and this one had me off in fairly short order, though Peter did get some photos first. But the Sherpas got the last word; they slew the yak and I believe we had him for supper.

"All work and no play....." We decided to climb Island Peak, or Imja Tse, a 20,305ft mountain separated from Everest only by the Lhotse-Nuptse ridge. We were joined by a lady climber that Peter had got to know; she had been climbing all alone in that area and he would have been highly critical of this if he had not known that she was a very experienced mountaineer. We trekked up a valley with a surprisingly long stretch of sand and then camped at the foot of the mountain overnight. We left Saila at the camp. I had hired some crampons from a Sherpa, though I was not entirely happy about them; they were twisted out of shape by previous use on large high altitude boots and tended to come loose.

At first we made good progress up the steep snow and ice slope and we were only a little short of the summit ridge when disaster struck. One of those pesky crampons came off completely, raced down the slope and disappeared into a deep crevasse. Without the ability to use the crampon's sharp points to dig into the ice, there was a severe risk that I would follow it all the way down. I only survived because of my expert help. First they belayed me up to the summit ridge where we re-grouped. Then, in the best mountaineering tradition, they gave up their own opportunity of reaching the summit to help me down to our camp. Perhaps one of my least enjoyable and most ignominious days in the mountains!

Saila and I had a good scramble on the flanks of Mount Ama Dablam, one of the most striking of the Khumbhu peaks. We got to a point quite high on one of the ridges before realising that it would be suicidal to go higher without better equipment—and more experienced companions! Saila said he had a headache because of the wind, but I believe he actually had early benign acute mountain sickness.

It was great trip generally, but there were a couple of bad days on the way down. First I had a very severe, though fortunately quite short, episode of diarrhoea and vomiting. Possibly the yak's revenge! We were close to the Japanese hotel at Syangboche. This had recently been built and had its own airstrip. That it was not a success was due to the failure to realise that, at 12,400ft, the danger to un-acclimatised people arriving by air was considerable. Even though they provided oxygen in the bedrooms, it was not a pleasant experience. (I am told that nowadays people go up for breakfast and a good view and return soon after.) Anyway, the manager was very happy to let me use a room for the night; I don't think there were any other visitors.

Then, when we got to Lukla, we found that all flights had been cancelled because of bad weather in Kathmandu. So there was a large crowd of tourists getting more and more hungry as supplies dwindled and our return was delayed. When planes did arrive from Kathmandu, they brought supplies of bread for the stranded visitors.

More Hillary Tales

Following our first meeting at Khunde Hospital, I saw quite a bit of Ed Hillary over the years. He suffered a great tragedy when the plane carrying his first wife and daughter crashed after take-off at Kathmandu Airport on a flight to join him in Paphlu in the southern (Solu) part of the Solu Khumbhu District.

This must have been in his mind when we went to the airport together on a later occasion. His son, Peter, was a well-known climber in his own right and had gone to the Khumbhu with four friends from New Zealand to climb Mount Ama Dablam. An urgent message arrived saying that an avalanche had swept away all four New Zealanders. Two had died and two were injured and being helicoptered to Kathmandu. But as we went to meet them, Ed did not know if Peter was one of the survivors or one of the dead. However father and son were duly re-united in a low key fashion; neither of them was given to overt emotion. We took Peter to Shanta Bhawan, where he again showed remarkable stoicism. As the surgeon poked and moved his various limbs asking "Does that hurt?" Peter merely grunted "Yeah", with no signs of distress. He had, I think, 13 fractures!

Ed was very averse to publicity, especially if he was admitted to hospital. He had a medical problem on one occasion and wanted to be anonymous, so we had in the ward a certain Mr Hill!

He was appointed the High Commissioner of New Zealand to India, based in New Delhi and at the same time Ambassador to Nepal. As was customary, on each visit he would host a drinks party in a Kathmandu hotel to which the great and the good were invited (as well as me and a number of Sherpas and climbing friends!) When the smarter set had departed, Hillary hilarity and Sherpa dancing continued late into the night.

Ed was admitted to Patan Hospital several years after I had left it. In spite of being really quite sick, he apparently consented to be the guest of honour at the opening of the new Children's Ward and made the expected celebrity contribution.

It is said that when Hillary and Tensing were asked how they felt on the summit of Everest, Hillary said "Bloody good!" and Tensing said "I thought of god and his greatness". As you might expect, I thought Tensing's comment was the more inspiring, but none the less Ed Hillary was a great man.

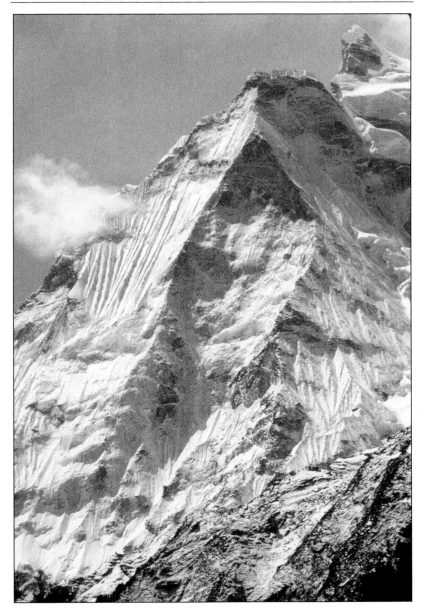

The Steep Slopes of Mt Ama Dablam. Photo: Dr Gerry Hankins

The Yak in the Fridge.

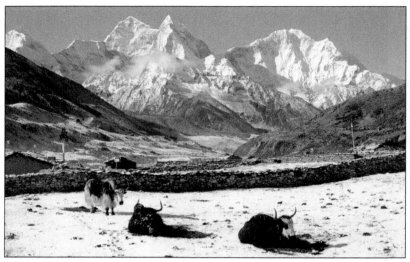

Yaks beneath Mts. Kangtega and Thamaserkhu. Photo: Dr Gerry Hankins

Well, to be honest, it was only the heart of a yak and part of its lung, but still Angela was not best pleased! I had got involved in a research project with Professor Donald Heath of the Pathology Department in the University of Liverpool and one of his team, David Williams. Donald had done a good deal of work on high altitude in the Andes and written a book 'Man at High Altitude' in which he quoted work on the llama, alpaca and other Andean high altitude animals. He was keen to do some studies on the Himalayan yak and asked me to collaborate. My major contribution was to obtain a specimen of yak heart and lung. This I did through Sherpa friends as yaks only live at high altitude. Thus it was that I became author in 1984, with Donald and David, of a paper on "The Pulmonary Arteries of the Yak", an element of my CV that has caused a certain amount of merriment among my medical friends. (Heath D, Williams D, Dickinson J, 1984)

I had to package and seal these gory remains and take them to the airport to see them through the Customs process. It took a fair amount of explaining, but none of the Customs Officers seemed to have a liking for the idea of opening the packages for inspection!

[*Angela says:* I was very pleased to see the plane depart and the bits of yak with it!]

For those who understand these things, we showed that the yak has evolved to lose a mechanism called Hypoxic Arteriolar Vasoconstriction in its lungs. This is a mechanism in most of the human race and other mammals to regulate blood supply to the lungs in such a way that blood is directed away from alveoli (lung units) that do not contain air (and therefore oxygen) at any given time. This is a considerable advantage at sea level because otherwise this blood would be shunted through the lungs without picking up any oxygen. The problem with it at high altitude is that all parts of the lungs contain blood with lower oxygen levels, more or less equally. There is no need to redistribute the blood flow and constriction of the blood vessels leading to the lungs simply increases the pressure in the pulmonary artery and makes the heart work harder.

If low altitude cattle are taken to live at high altitude, they develop this high pressure and, helped by a thickening of the blood, it leads to heart failure and death. This is called Brisket Disease, because the skin over the chest becomes swollen with excess fluid, which is a sign of heart failure in cattle.

Do humans get this? Yes; people in the Andes suffer from a similar condition in middle age called Chronic Mountain Sickness. However, Tibetans and Sherpas in the Himalaya do not get this disease and more recent research has shown that they have a much smaller increase in pulmonary artery pressure and also their blood is less thick. So they have this evolutionary adaptation in common with their yaks.

My apologies for inflicting this science on you if it's not your interest, but it is a nice little biological question solved in a satisfactory way. (You will see that I am not one of those Christians who do not believe in evolution.) I enjoyed all this, though I was clearly guilty of abuse of the domestic fridge!

Chapter 11.

A Doctor is a Teacher!

People are sometimes surprised to learn that the word 'doctor' comes from a Latin verb meaning to teach. I suppose there was a progression from teacher to learned man to natural philosopher to someone with the knowledge to deal with illness. So now a doctor is a medical doctor by default and any other kind needs to be explained; PhD, for instance. Not that the qualifying degree in UK and many other countries is an academic doctorate; mostly it is a Bachelor's degree in Medicine and Surgery, something like MB BS, though there are lots of variants. I particularly like the Irish one which also includes BAO; Bachelor of the Art of Obstetrics! In North America, the basic qualification is an MD, though it is not a doctorate in the academic sense.

Several other surprises come in the Hippocratic Oath, which is not in fact taken by medical doctors any more, though there are more modern variations. I like the original second paragraph:

"To consider dear to me, as my parents, him who taught me this art; to live in common with him and, if necessary, to share my goods with him; To look upon his children as my own brothers, to teach them this art; and that by my teaching, I will impart a knowledge of this art to my own sons, and to my teacher's sons, and to disciples bound by an indenture and oath according to the medical laws, and no others."

For one thing, it amuses me to point out to my students that the Oath would require them to share their goods with me to keep me in my old age. They don't seem impressed by this, somehow! But, more seriously, there is an obligation to pass on the "art" to others.

In Nepal, I started by giving classes to student nurses as well as trying to teach them things at the bedside wherever possible. If I was lucky enough to have a House Physician (junior doctor, resident, intern) I would teach him (or occasionally her) as well. Gradually, a few expatriate medical students would learn about Shanta Bhawan and come to us for electives. In the mid-70s, I was asked to teach young men training to be Health Assistants, paramedicals intended to work in District Hospitals and Health Posts. Mostly, this would be practical training in clinical skills on the wards at Shanta Bhawan. I also helped train Village Health Assistants, mostly women this time, who were to work at village community level. They were generally educated to a very low level, so the teaching was necessarily practical and not at all academic. This is how 'doctor' quickly became ' teacher'.

The First Medical School in Nepal

Some of the material in the remaining sections of this chapter is also to be found in Appendix I, an article that I wrote for the British Medical Journal in 1984.

The project to develop a Medical School in Nepal began in the mid-70s and, as a result of my teaching activities, I was asked to be involved with people from the Nepal government, World Health Organisation and others in planning the new Medical School at the grandly-named Institute of Medicine of Tribhuwan University in Maharajganj in the north of Kathmandu. This excited me, and I hoped to have the opportunity of teaching medicine and clinical skills to the first home-grown doctors, since, up to that point, most Nepalese doctors were trained in India. However as the opening approached in 1978 it was obvious that Nepalese doctors wanted the positions of Lecturer, Reader and Professor in Medicine and I rather bowed out of the process.

Eventually the day of the inaugural tea party arrived and I was invited to attend. Naturally I wanted an update on progress and was told that plans were reasonably well developed, but they were lacking in basic science teachers, especially for Anatomy and Physiology. Now I happened to have a Master's degree in Animal Physiology from

Oxford, and I had always seen physiology as an important basis for clinical medicine. 'Clinical Physiology' by Campbell, Dickinson and Slater had always been one of my faithful textbooks. (The Dickinson had nothing to do with me, but Moran Campbell became a friend as I have described in a different context).

One of my friends at Shanta Bhawan, Paul Spivey, was already working with IoM to develop a course for pharmacists. The UMN Health Services Director, Carl Friedericks, who had an academic background as Professor of Public Health in the USA, was supportive of the medical school project. So after consultation and agreement from Carl, I offered my services for the physiology course.

This was to be in addition to my work at the hospital. I found a certain amount of resistance among my colleagues to this additional appointment as it meant someone would have to cover my duties for some of the time. Then it became apparent that I was to be the only member of the physiology department and that it fell to me to draw up a curriculum and design the entire course. Fortunately, one of the innovative aspects of the course was that it began with a whole nine months in which the students studied public health and spent time in village communities. This allowed time to do some detailed planning.

Limited Facilities

Now I have to explain what I meant by 'the grandly- named Institute of Medicine of Tribhuwan University'. The University was well-established by this time, but the IoM was in a couple of blocks of simple buildings close to the Kanti Children's Hospital. (This was indeed 'to the North of Kathmandu' of the entirely fictional poem about the One-Eyed Yellow Idol, but had nothing to do with it!)

No Teaching Hospital existed then, though it was completed around 1986 along the lines of Shanta Bhawan's replacement, Patan Hospital. The Japanese architects deliberately copied many of the features of the building. Meanwhile, as students came to the clinical parts of their course, they were assigned to busy hospitals where heavy service commitments made it hard for doctors to give them the necessary attention.

In the simple buildings, there were limited supplies of water and electricity and nothing in the way of teaching and learning aids.

Staff worked in dusty offices without significant office equipment. The classrooms had ancient blackboards on which the chalk left very little mark at all. So when it came to teaching physiology I depended upon buying large sheets of cartridge paper and some marker pens, pinning diagrams to the walls and rushing madly from one to another trying to illustrate physiological principles and processes. When it eventually came into my life as a medical teacher at a different medical school, PowerPoint was a huge relief!

An innovative Course

There were some interesting innovations in the course, designed to meet the requirements of the country's medical need.

Firstly, all the students were selected only from those who had worked in the Health Services. Examples were former Health Assistants, Pharmacists, Radiographers, Laboratory Technicians, Nurses and traditional (Ayurvedic) practitioners. In the first batch, there were only 22 students and the facilities could not have coped with more. Unfortunately in my opinion, this excellent philosophy was changed after a few years to select only from those who had passed the '10 + 2' level of education. This doubtless reflected the upgraded academic standards of the University as a whole, but it meant that students no longer had experience of working in the Health Services and the sense of serving patients that such experience could bring.

Secondly, their future roles were defined under three headings, as follows:

1. A clinical role to save life, to restore health and rehabilitate by providing medical care in a District Hospital.
2. A preventive role in maternal and child health, environmental health, health education, communicable disease control and school health.
3. An administrative role, collecting and updating appropriate demographic and epidemiological data, planning and implementing comprehensive health care in the district, functioning as leader, and ensuring the effective functioning of the health care team in the district.

Would any of today's medical graduates in the UK feel prepared to take on such varied roles after four years plus a hospital internship? The emphasis on community health aspects was the reason why the first nine months were spent in community-based learning, and this continued throughout the course.

Thirdly, there was an attempt at integrated, system-based learning of basic medical sciences. This was then in the early stages of development in Medical Schools such as Dundee in Scotland and McMaster in Canada. Lip service was given to Problem Based Learning, but this was never really achieved. However, as students worked on systems such as respiratory or cardiovascular, I, as the only clinician among the basic science staff, was able to give them practical demonstrations and some elementary clinical skills teaching at Shanta Bhawan. I really enjoyed this, and especially their eagerness to learn. I believe they valued this element of the course.

Physiology Teaching

I would like to describe something of my own efforts to develop a philosophy and curriculum for physiology (which tacitly included biochemistry). I wanted it to be a practical subject, closely allied to the practice of medicine, rather than an academic discipline. To this end, I renamed it Clinical Physiology to emphasise its importance in understanding clinical work. I organised little in the way of traditional 'physiology practicals', partly because there was no apparatus to do them, but also because I believed there was more to be learnt from using eyes, ears, hands and the simple equipment that would be available in a District Hospital. So, for example, I would have the students run around a field and make observations on each other. They would measure heart rate, respiratory rate and blood pressure and observe changes in the skin such as sweating and dilatation of blood vessels.

The Physiology Department (ie me!) had no laboratory equipment and limited access to library books. I selected a physiology textbook which was quite simple and available and had originally been written for nurses. This may seem un-ambitious, but I was keen that these students, with their limited English, should learn the basics well and build upon that rather than attempt large and complicated tomes from the beginning.

Delays

Compared to westerners, the Nepalese have a casual attitude to time and timetables. There was no fixed University Calendar in those early days. Students would be released when the term's work was finished, went to their homes (which might well be far away in the hills) and then they would return—when they returned! Without fixed terms, it was hard to complete the curriculum in the time originally envisaged. This was responsible for a delay of the best part of a year for the first batch. On top of this were frequent student agitations for various reasons, many political. As a result of this, we lost another 18 months. Instead of four years, they graduated after six and a half years.

It was not that the medical students wanted to take part in the various strikes; on the contrary, they were highly motivated to get on and finish their course. The only problem was that they liable to get beaten up if they attended classes! I remember giving a class when students from other faculties descended on the classroom and demanded that the students leave at once. I am sad to say they capitulated without a struggle, whereas I was spitting mad.

Incidentally on other occasions when students have a grievance against the University, they often padlock the offices of the Dean and other officers. A simple fellow like me would say that the authorities should simply cut off the padlock, but it seems that the philosophy in Nepal is different; the padlock belongs to someone else so it should not be cut off without their permission. I admit I never really got my head around this.

Many of the strikes in the early 80s were part of a general upheaval which led to the re-definition of the monarchy as a constitutional one, and many years later to the overthrow of the monarchy altogether. It could be said that it was part of a process of developing democracy and that the sacrifices were worthwhile. As someone who was trying to help the training of much-needed medical manpower, I have to say that I did not see it in that light then, and have not fully accepted it now. And Nepal is still struggling over the true meaning of democracy. Groups still make their views and protests known by violence, strikes, lockouts and the '*bandh*' or shut down of roads, shops and businesses.

Final examinations

Among all these limitations and upheavals, I had the privilege of teaching physiology to the first two years of the first MB BS course to be run in Nepal. I was later designated 'Professor', but I was still the only member of the Physiology Department! People would ask if the graduates would be real doctors and if their medical degrees would be accepted in other countries. In spite of all our limitations, I am pleased and proud to say that the course was a success. In April 1984, the results of the final examinations for the first batch were announced. Twelve succeeded and the remainder passed on re-take. I was present at some of the clinical and oral examinations. Generally the students showed a high standard of history-taking, physical examination and diagnosis, even though they struggled because the exams were in English. There were three external examiners. One, an Indian, asked if he could take the successful students back to India with him (No!) and a Canadian said that they compared favourably with his students at home.

I have met up with many old students over the years and most have done very well. One has been responsible for establishing two different medical schools in Nepal (and invited his old physiology teacher to teach students of his own). Another has become a well-known plastic surgeon and gives many hours of community service, such as repairing hare lips in rural surgical camps. Another became doctor to the British Gurkhas and later to the Nepalese element of the forces of the Sultan of Brunei. Another became a Professor of Anatomy. Yet another held high office in the Nepal Medical Association. Many obtained postgraduate qualifications, some in western countries.

Physiology, Frogs and a Politician

I have explained my attitude to 'Physiology Practicals'. However I came under quite a lot of pressure to arrange the sort of experiments that had been done for ever in other medical schools. Finally I agreed to set up frog nerve-muscle preparations. This bit is not for the squeamish, I'm afraid! The frog has its brain destroyed by 'pithing', the passing of a needle through the back of the neck into the brain.

One of its large leg muscles is then dissected out complete with the nerve that supplies it. This is all kept moist as far as possible and mounted on a stand so that electrical impulses can be applied to the nerve (or the muscle). One end of the muscle is connected to a stylus that writes on a revolving drum so that the responses to different strengths and patterns of stimulus can be recorded. It is traditional, interesting and quite informative.

Praying that the electricity would not be off that day, I planned an afternoon of nerve-muscle experiments with my students. Now normal physiology departments will ask their Lab Technician to contact the biological supply agency to obtain the necessary number of frogs and he would probably set up some of the experiments in advance, demonstrating the techniques to the students when they arrive. In our case there was no Lab Tech and no biological supply agency. As it happened, our daughter was a pre-medical student at the time and quite interested and we knew from the loud croaking in the evenings that the local ponds had a large frog population. So we set off after dark on my little motor bike and found some suitable ponds. One of us directed the headlight of the motor bike and the other guddled about in the ponds trying to catch the frogs. This was tricky and quite hilarious, but we managed to capture a fair number and put them in tins (which had originally held Plaster of Paris as I remember).

Next day both of us climbed onto the bike again with the live frogs in their tins and a lot of equipment that I had been given during a period spent picking the brains of some kind folk in the physiology department of Glasgow University. Imagine us festooned with tins of frogs, bags and rucksacks! Thus we wobbled our way to the Institute of Medicine well in time to get everything set up for the students at 2 pm. We were delighted to find that everything worked as it should and eagerly awaited the arrival of the class. At 2 pm, there was no-one there. Still no-one at 2.30 or 3 pm. Finally, about 3.30 pm a lone emissary turned up to explain that a prominent opposition politician had died and they felt it their duty to march in the procession to show their sympathy.

As we wearily disposed of the drying shreds of nerve and muscle and the corpses that had originally contained them (and then released the few remaining live frogs) I concluded that there had been nothing wrong with my original policy on practicals and resolved that, whatever other predators may raid their ponds, the frogs of Kathmandu would henceforth have nothing to fear from me. [See Chapter 3 for Mary's account of this]

In spite of this discouragement in terms of practical experiments, I found a great deal of inspiration in teaching physiology; the way the human body works. I was constantly reminded of the Biblical line "We are fearfully and wonderfully made" as I taught how the body adjusts to a whole variety of environmental challenges and demands such as exercise and pregnancy. Though Professor Richard Dawkins and others see science as supplanting faith, I have always seen it as exactly the reverse. It is a privilege to see the handiwork of the Creator in the amazing mechanisms of the bodies he has given us. Though I felt unable to testify to this spiritual aspect in classes and writings because of our mission agreement with government, I did write a series in the Medical School Journal which I entitled 'Wonderland of Physiology'. In this, I sought to express my sense of wonder at the interlocking mechanisms that allow us to survive and thrive and respond to our environment. When Dr Arjun Karki, who had been one of my students, later established the Medical School at Patan Hospital, he asked me to re-create at least the spirit of this series in a lecture for his own students.

With all the delays and limitations, this was a time of frustration, but also of great satisfaction. Though I always wanted to go on seeing patients, I saw my life developing along the paths of academe; teaching, following up my research interests, especially in high altitude physiology and mountain sickness and working on a physiology textbook specifically for Nepal that I thought was needed. It didn't happen this way, and the reason will be revealed in the next chapter.

Chapter 12.

Patan Hospital

he old Rana palace at Shanta Bhawan served as a hospital from 1956 to 1983. However, in the late 70s, United Mission to Nepal began to think about replacing it with a purpose-built hospital. One Medical Superintendent, asked how long the old building could stand, replied that it would depend how many layers of paint could be applied! (I should state that it was still standing and in use as a school until it was damaged by the earthquake of April 2015.) Another reason was that it was off the main roads, and especially the bus routes which were being established quickly as the road system gradually improved.

The site selected was at Lagankhel in Patan, a point at which several important roads converge, bringing buses and traffic from the Lalitpur District, one of the three in the Kathmandu Valley. Money was raised, predominantly from Germany, to build the new hospital, plans were drawn up and building began. [*Angela says:* It was being talked about when we arrived in 1969. It finally opened in 1982.] His Majesty, King Birendra Bir Bikram Shah Dev, was invited to perform the Grand Opening in November 1982. This was fine, except that the hospital was by no means completed in time! As the opening approached, staff planning became urgent. An excellent American internist, Kathy Witherington, was rightly designated head of the Department of Medicine and I put my name forward as a part time consultant while I continued my role in the Medical School. I have to admit that I was quite disappointed when I was told that my services would not be required!

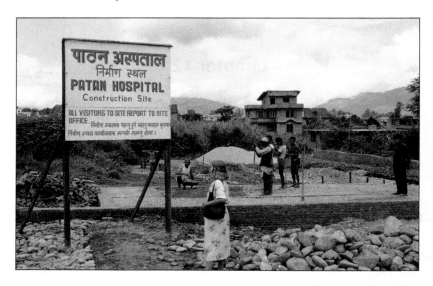

Patan Hospital: the Building Site. Photo: Dr Gerry Hankins

However, circumstances conspired to bring about an entirely different outcome and the time has come to narrate them. Del Haug was a Canadian doctor who had done a very good job as the Medical Superintendent of the UMN hospital at Tansen in the West. He had long been chosen to assume the same role at the new hospital.

Angela (forgive the digression, but it is relevant) was organising the orientation course for new UMN workers and we both went with the group to spend a weekend in Dhulikhel (17 miles to the east). She was leading a long walk through the hills, when there was an unexpected shower causing her to slip on a steep path and fracture her fibula. Bravely, she walked for the remaining three hours on this spiral fracture. Back in Kathmandu she refused a plaster of Paris cast, but was told to keep her weight off the leg.

After a few days, I was called to Shanta Bhawan where Del, the designated Medical Director, was quite seriously ill. I found a cranial nerve palsy and after a few hours, evidence of meningitis. He had a brain abscess which was leaking pus into his cerebrospinal fluid.

This was an emergency that we could not cope with in Nepal, with no CT scanner anywhere in the country and limited neurosurgery. So he had to be flown urgently to Bangkok, complete with his wife and daughters. A Canadian anaesthetist was delegated to accompany him. However, with little more than an hour to go before take-off time, I got an urgent message to say that the Canadian did not feel he could cope with the responsibility of a severely ill medical patient and I was to go instead.

So you can imagine me hastily packing a few things, leaving Angela and dashing to the airport with my passport. I felt guilty about Angela, but in fact our good neighbours, Gerry and Alison Hankins, took very good care of her as her bone knitted itself.

Bangkok

In the end, many good things came out of my time in Bangkok, which lasted about a week. Most importantly, Del had a CT scan, the abscess was drained and he started on a long, but complete, process of recovery. The main mission representative of our mutual mission society, Michael Roemmele, 'happened' to be in Bangkok and was able to facilitate all the important financial arrangements for Del's treatment, his family and their later return to Canada. Yes, I saw this as God's provision.

Meanwhile I met up with a well-known Thai Respiratory Physician with whom I had previously had an interesting correspondence about sarcoidosis. He would not allow me to buy my own dinners, but took me each evening to a different fascinating Bangkok restaurant for dinners of different international flavours.

I was also able to contact David and Mary Warrell. David had been a brilliant fellow student with me at Oxford and was by this time Professor of Tropical Medicine there. He had set up a research unit in Bangkok, working on snakebite, malaria and rabies among other things. I spent some time in his unit, enjoying exposure to a much more sophisticated level of academic medicine than I was used to. Somehow, I didn't feel like using my Nepal title of 'Professor' in David's presence!

After about a week, Del's condition was improving steadily and I felt able to return to Nepal. He and his family were to go to Canada for what proved to be a long period of convalescence. He did eventually return to Nepal, though not to Patan Hospital.

Back in Nepal

Ironically for a man who had been told there was no place for him at Patan Hospital, I found myself asked, indeed expected, to take over as Medical Director! This was not based on my qualities or qualifications for the job, but on the unflattering fact that there was no-one else! As I was enjoying my role at the Medical School and had no administrative training or pretensions, I was very reluctant. Apart from loyalty to the mission, two main factors swayed my decision. One was that the political situation of the time was likely to result in the University and the Medical School being closed for an indefinite period, and indeed that proved to be so. (I had been planning to use the time to write the textbook that I have mentioned.) The other reason was that I had a very long-standing and close relationship with most of the Nepali staff that were to transfer from Shanta Bhawan. Rightly or wrongly, they were feeling insecure about the move for a variety of reasons, one having been that they were apprehensive about leadership from a Director that they did not know and who came from a hospital which had a very different nature. I concluded that I owed them an element of continuity, even though I knew that the character of the new hospital would have to be very different.

Patan Hospital

It was really only just before the Grand Opening that the planners released the name of the new hospital. I have to say that many felt that it was unimaginative, but it settled in reasonably quickly. However the local people called it *'Naya Shanta Bhawan'* or 'New Shanta Bhawan' for many years.

I should explain that Kathmandu and Patan are the Liverpool and Birkenhead of Nepal; two cities on opposite sides of a river. They are two of the three cities in the Kathmandu Valley and they are joined by a bridge over the Bagmati River. The third city is Bhaktapur about nine miles to the East. It was then separated by a good deal of agricultural land, but Kathmandu and Bhaktapur have since become more or less continuous.

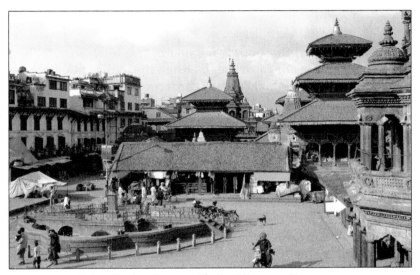

Patan Durbar Square. Photo: Maureen Newman

Patan was the main city and administrative centre of Lalitpur District, which extends south from the city to the edge of the Kathmandu Valley and beyond into the hills. Although in the opposite direction from the mighty Himalaya, these hills are as steep and rugged as the foothills to the north and the population of the district was of the order of 200,000 people. The intention was that the hospital would serve the preventive and curative medical needs of the District. To this end, it was agreed that Patan Hospital would replace the small Lalitpur Hospital, which was situated just the other side of the main road, together with the functions and responsibilities of the District Medical Officer.

The hospital was to be run by a Board consisting of representatives of the Government, Local Community and the mission. I'll have some comments about how this worked out later! The day-to-day administration was the responsibility of the Administrative Officer, Bir Bahadur Khawas, the Nursing Superintendent, Ruth Judd, and me as

Medical Director. Though by no means always in agreement, I believe we worked well together in a difficult and sometimes tense situation.

Hospital or Building Site?

As I explained, the Grand Opening of the New Hospital had been arranged a year in advance to ensure the participation of King Birendra. Though the building was far from finished, the Opening went ahead in November 1982.

I was not responsible for the hospital, though, until the beginning of January 1983, that is, a couple of months later. Up to that point, the Medical Director of Shanta Bhawan, Dr Archie Fletcher, took the responsibility before he retired. As I have said, much building work remained to be done, though many parts of the basic structure were spruced up to look convincing for the Royal Visit.

Only after I took over were we ready to begin transferring services from Shanta Bhawan. Initially, inpatients stayed at Shanta Bhawan and its operating theatre remained in use, but outpatients were seen at Patan. The rooms in the new Out Patient Department were still without doors and many other fittings, but services were just about possible. The laboratory came to Patan, but the x ray and dental departments and the kitchen remained at Shanta Bhawan. One of the hardest things was that staff quarters were far from ready and the nursing staff in particular had to be bussed about a mile and a half from Shanta Bhawan and back. The pharmacy, social services, cashiers and administrative staff had to divide up and perform their functions in both places.

The building boss was Martyn Thomas and it was very helpful that we were good friends. (You may recall that he got engaged to be married in our house.) He was even my patient on occasion. As a conscientious building engineer, he was very protective of his side of the project as opposed to my side, the working hospital. One thing he didn't appreciate at all was various members of the hospital staff approaching him to ask for changes in the plans for their own departments. He was understandably unwilling to tamper with the architect's plans as he went along. So he made it a rule that all requests and co-ordination went through me and it became my job and pleasure to join him and his international team for coffee each morning. This enabled us to discuss issues informally. He also had various barriers erected to Separate the working hospital from the building project. Though this got quite complicated, and some of the hospital folk were inclined to take offence, I'm sure in retrospect it was the right policy and we came to respect one another's views more and more.

None the less, I'm sure you can imagine the tensions that developed at times, for example when carpenters came into offices and clinics to install doors and window fittings. Of course we were grateful for these things, but the disruptions could be frustrating.

Returning to the question of changing the plans; department heads at Shanta Bhawan had been canvassed quite properly 4-5 years before about the needs of their departments in terms of space, rooms, equipment, power and light and so on. This was the basis for the architect's plans. But people come and go; by 1983 many of the original department heads had been replaced by others, whose ideas were often different. In no department was this more of a problem than in the Dental Department. The current dentist had strong views and, for him, the planned department was entirely inadequate. Martyn dug in his heels and refused to change. Higher authorities became involved and it was a long time before it was all resolved with concessions on both sides and a certain amount of unseemly ill feeling. The Dental Department was, I think, the last to move from Shanta Bhawan. Though I tried to placate and mediate, this was a time when I had major regrets about accepting the post.

The building was four stories high and much longer than it was wide. Out patients, offices, laundry and housekeeping, kitchen, library and maintenance were all on the ground floor. Surgery and theatres were on the first floor and medicine and obstetrics and gynaecology on the second. Paediatrics and private patients were to have been on the top floor, but unfortunately there had been a funding shortfall and the use of the top floor was put on hold. A temporary Children's Ward was created on the ground floor behind the laboratory, physiotherapy and X-ray Department, but it was much smaller than we really needed.

There was to have been a separate block of staff quarters, but the building of this had not even started. The only solution was to construct nurses' rooms in the shell of the top floor.

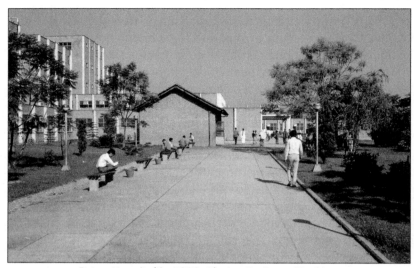

Patan Hospital in 1986. Photo: Dr Gerry Hankins

Though much of the equipment was ready when the hospital started, some was delayed. This was particularly true of the X-ray machines, which had to be imported from India and installed by Indian engineers.

I fear this recounting of difficulties and frustrations may become tedious. I have already described the difficulties of starting a Medical School from scratch in Nepal, now it is the turn of the hospital. I don't want to hold anyone to account over these problems; delays and cost overruns are far from rare in my own country. However it became very clear to me that it would have been far better to have waited at least a year to enable many more of the construction elements to be completed and all equipment installed. I'm sure Martyn felt the same and would have been happy to get on with the task without my trying to run a hospital at the same time.

Philosophy of Patan Hospital

PH was not meant to be 'New Shanta Bhawan'. The philosophy was to be quite different. First it was to be a District Hospital according to the government system. However it was also to provide the 138 beds that were lost at Shanta Bhawan. This would make it some 10 times the size of most District Hospitals. The staff of the existing Lalitpur District Hospital was to be transferred to PH, including the District Medical Officer who was responsible for public health and performing autopsies, which was a government requirement. We were to inherit the old hospital building and I will return to this later.

The status as a District Hospital meant that the services were to be those of basic secondary care and not include any specialties. This was a problem for my surgeon friend Gerry Hankins; it meant that the very good Nepali Orthopaedic Surgeon who had been working at Shanta Bhawan could not transfer to the PH staff. Orthopaedics and trauma would have to be managed by general surgeons as best they could.

As I mentioned, the Hospital Board was to consist of representatives from the government, the local community and the mission. In the first instance, the government and community folk took the attitude that UMN had been running hospitals for years and they could manage the new hospital. In fact it was extremely difficult to arrange Board meetings at a time when they could attend, especially the Ministry of Health representative who seemed to us to be a crucial member. With time, however this changed and local politics was strengthened in the country generally. Unfortunately, this brought in a number of issues more relevant to the re-election of the official than to patient care and services to the community. I am afraid I lost a number of battles at Board meetings, including my attempt to increase the number of doctors and another to accelerate the building of a bigger and better Children's Ward. With nearly half the population of the country being under 15 years of age, it seemed to me that we needed a proportionately larger number of beds and facilities for children.

I struggled with the question "Who are the Community?" It seemed of central importance that we should provide the services that the 'Community' wanted, but who should we be listening to? There were the wealthy business and professional people, who would want more private care and more specialism, the very poor, who generally had no voice but were in need of free or very inexpensive care and a range of folk in between, belonging to a variety of castes and trades. Almost nobody had any real vision for preventive medicine; they thought a hospital was for curing the sick. Our philosophy, however, laid stress on promotive and preventive medicine, as a result of which the Community Development and Health Project (CDHP) was housed on the hospital site.

In the interests of providing cheap, basic medical care, we developed a technique that had been tested in the last few years at Shanta Bhawan. All new outpatients were initially seen by paramedicals, Health Assistants, who were specially trained and supervised by an American Family Practitioner and his colleagues. Anyone they could not treat was referred to a generalist doctor and possibly then to a physician, surgeon or gynaecologist. Though they were sometimes disparagingly termed 'sorters' these Health Assistants actually did a very good job and my American colleague, Bob Gsellman, worked out that they could satisfactorily manage some 80% of the patients that came to them. [*Mary says:* I did my elective in Patan Hospital, and worked alongside one of the health assistants there. They worked very much as GPs and more; they knew an astonishing amount. They could hear subtleties of heart and lung sounds through a stethoscope in a room of 100 noisy patients and relatives. I still have total respect for the skills of Bishnu, who I was shadowing, now head of the dental department at PH.]

Sadly in my view, and after my time at PH, this system was abolished as a result of pressure from influential patients who wanted to be seen by 'proper doctors' from the beginning. Of course, I was not involved in this, but my questions would have been "Who do we listen to?" and "Whose interests are best served by the change?"

Primary Care in the Hospital

CDHP provided clinics in various villages in the District, some well beyond the edge of the Valley. We used to provide doctors to help with this, but there were always tensions arising from the conflicting demands of huge patient numbers in the hospitals and fewer in the clinics, but with the opportunities for preventive and promotive care.

We set up a referral system from village clinics in which referred patients came with a letter and were fast-tracked to a suitable doctor without paying a registration fee. They were then sent back with a letter. (This was in a country which then had no real notion of referring patients and sharing information about them.) We also experimented with a health insurance system which had a certain limited success, though naturally people were reluctant to pay the premiums.

This may not seem a great deal of progress, but I got a big surprise one day; two really. Up to then any international phone calls had to come through the central post office in the shadow of Bhim Sen Tower in the centre of Kathmandu. This always involved long waits. But I picked up the phone in my office at PH to find that I had a call from the World Health Organisation in Geneva. Apparently someone had told them about our efforts in the primary care arena and I was invited to Geneva to act as a WHO consultant in the production of a publication on Primary Care in the Hospital. I protested that we were merely feeling our way and that surely other groups had more to share than we did, but they insisted. So I produced some written materials and eventually went to Geneva for a few days and contributed to the report. (WHO, 1987)

I think, with very little exaggeration, I was paid more for those few days than I received as a mission allowance to support me and my family for the entire year.

Visiting a remote area

I was occasionally able to make visits to the CDHP clinics. On one memorable occasion, I was able to take Angela with me to villages in Southern Lalitpur, well beyond the edge of the Kathmandu Valley. I have mentioned that these hills, though in the opposite direction to the main Himalayan range, are still very rugged and we found to our cost just how tough walking in them may be. We were taken by a 4WD vehicle to the edge of the valley and walked on to a Health Post where we were had been assured that we would be able to get *daal bhat*, the standard Nepali meal. However this proved not to be the case. Hungry, we pressed on down into a valley, and then up through the hills to our destination, another Health Post on a high ridge. It was May and hot; the temperature well into the 30s C. There were few sources of drinkable water and it was a long climb. I followed my hot weather trekking practice of soaking my hat in any available water, drinkable or not, and hoping that the sun would evaporate that water instead of my sweat. In spite of that, even I, who had done a good deal of hard trekking, had to flop down beside the trail to recover before I could go on. I do not remember ever having been so weary and suppose the lack of food had something to do with it. Angela was not carrying a load, but she very creditably plodded on through the heat.

Arriving at last we were able to slake our thirst, but it was still a long time before our hosts prepared a *daal-bhat* meal for us. Next day, recovered, we pressed on to the Health Post at Ashrang. There I saw quite a large number of patients, including a woman with a huge abscess of her breast. I'm no surgeon, but it was relatively simple to incise and drain this under local anaesthetic. [*Angela says:* I don't remember any anaesthetic and she cried blue murder.] I was able to encourage and teach the Auxiliary Nurse Midwives who worked in this isolated place.

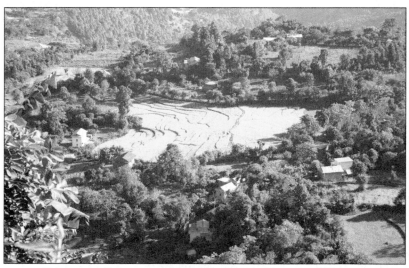

Eking out a living among the hills. Photo: Maureen Newman.

The next day included a visit that was one of the most emotional in our experience. We were taken to a small, dark hovel with a tiny patch of stony land, the home of a man and woman and their children. The wife and all the children had TB and it was apparent that it had become resistant to treatment. As we squatted in that dark, depressing place, Angela felt that death was there as a presence with us. [*Angela says:* we both cried.] She later made arrangements for supplies of '*sarbottam pitho*' or super flour, to be delivered to them regularly to help with the obvious malnutrition of the children However we later heard that wife and children all died, one of the children after returning from a period of care by Mother Theresa's Sisters in Kathmandu.

Not very long after our visit, Princess Diana was taken to the same area by helicopter and she must have come across similar heart-rending scenes. All the British newspapers showed the inevitable photos of her in Southern Lalitpur, together with her heartfelt "I will never complain again!"

Patan Hospital Staff

As I have already mentioned, the agreement between UMN and the government provided for the transfer of the government staff of the old District Hospital to PH. They clearly had mixed feelings. On the one hand, they were paid a good deal more, but on the other, more was expected of them. They worked longer hours and some were needed for emergency duties. In some cases, this would have interfered with other jobs that they may have had on the side and with private practice for the doctors. It was not easy for them to accept the authority of the officers of Patan Hospital; Medical Director, Nursing Superintendent and Administrative Officer. It took them time to adapt to our 'Shanta Bhawan' working practices; arriving on time, leaving on time (or later if required) and taking defined tea and meal breaks.

It was also a time of upheaval for the staff members who had come from Shanta Bhawan. For many, the old building had been home, as well as place of employment, and they had brought up their children on the premises. They had great affection for it. Many needed to rent, buy or build houses of their own. Ultimately this proved greatly to their advantage; they purchased land and built houses with some help from the hospital Provident Fund and the subsequent development of Kathmandu caused the land to increase greatly in value. As for the hospital work, the new environment was different and, though it carried promise of better things when the building was complete, it was meanwhile harder to adapt and work in it.

It was a help for doctors when I arranged for them to be paid over-time for emergency and on call duty. It may seem strange that this was an innovation! I am afraid I caused a headache for Bir Bahadur and others involved in balancing the budget, but we all believed it necessary in the interests of justice.

Staff quarters were a major problem. Initially workers were bussed from Shanta Bhawan and, after a while, rooms for nurses were improvised in the shell of the top floor. We had been promised the use of the former Lalitpur District Hospital building in the government-mission agreement. This held the promise of use for accommodating our staff. I visited it and requested the Ministry of Health to hand it over on several occasions. I met with a typical stonewall; absolutely no response. Then, after nearly a year, I spotted a newly-erected notice board outside the site saying "Mental Hospital". I do not know why the government chose to ignore an item in its own agreement, but I suppose we have all come to expect that governments make decisions that are opaque to the rest of us. I was never given an explanation and it remains a government mental hospital to this day.

Edging towards maturity

Gradually, things looked up. We were able to move inpatients and start doing surgery and delivering babies. The X-ray equipment was finally installed and the department moved. The Dental Department was the last of the clinical departments to be completed. Though outpatient numbers were low at first in comparison with Shanta Bhawan, they gradually picked up. The Emergency Department started to function well. CDHP moved into their block and began to work out of PH.

Three big electricity generators were installed with the capacity to take over automatically when the city supply failed. First one block of staff quarters was finished, then another.

Water was a big problem, as it usually is in Nepal. The city supply was inadequate and so we wanted a reliable deep well. A Chinese firm had dug several of these in the Kathmandu Valley and claimed that they had never failed to find water. I happened to have a Mandarin-speaking colleague working part time as my Secretary and she proved invaluable in communicating with the Chinese. In spite of all this, they failed to find deep, clean water for us. They drilled at several places and found water near the surface, so we were able to use these relatively shallow wells and their impure water for toilets, cleaning, laundry and so on. This was a help.

A Royal Visitor

Queen Aishwarya had taken to making surprise visits to public institutions to check if the officials were at their posts and doing their jobs. Several had been caught out and shamed. We didn't think Patan Hospital was likely to be on her list, and we didn't have anything to hide, so we weren't worried. Unfortunately, she came late on a Wednesday morning. On Wednesdays, the outpatient department was closed and the time was used for staff training. Almost the first thing she saw was a large group of doctors sitting in a circle in the sun outside the hospital! (It was winter, so that was the warmest place to sit.) In fact, they were having a teaching session on TB, led by one of the more junior doctors. As TB was one of my specialities, I had missed the session to avoid embarrassing him and gone home for an early lunch. No outpatients, doctors sitting around, Medical Director absent! Not a good first impression!

The hospital receptionist was flustered. Normally, very high forms of words are used for the Royal Family, but these deserted her when she phoned me urgently to say simply and breathlessly in Nepali "Queen came!" I was very close and got to the hospital quickly to find the Queen going round the wards with a train of followers, including a film crew from the recently-established Nepal Television. So the evening news included shots of me panting up to the Queen and trying to explain the situation on a Wednesday. She was distinctly cool to start with, but she apparently went away satisfied with my explanations.

Later Development

Gradually, and increasingly after my time, the government and local community (now really meaning local politicians) took over more responsibility for the decisions of the Hospital Board. UMN, keen to reduce its involvement in 'institutions', began to withdraw from the Board. When I left in 1986, with my recommendation, Bir

Bahadur was appointed as the Chief Executive Officer of the hospital; the Admin Officer rather than the Medical Director taking the overall responsibility. He did this extremely well for many years until his retirement. Health Assistants were replaced by doctors in OPD.

I will not try to record the detailed growth of the hospital, but it added a Children's Ward and an Orthopaedic Unit and later a very large, modern Obstetrics and Gynaecology wing. Amazingly for those of us who had come from Shanta Bhawan and the 'old days', it features central heating, air conditioning and an underground car park. This also allowed the opening of a Neonatal Intensive Care Unit. I had struggled to get the Board to agree to increase the number of doctors from 18, but I noted that it increased in later years to 50. In 2014 I was told there were 95 specialist level doctors and 85 at Resident level, giving a total of 180. (Some of the specialists, at least, are part time.) There are 300 nurses. The total bed number, originally officially 138 but less than that during the completion of the building, has now reached 450.

I was especially pleased about the opening of the Patan Academy of Health Sciences in 2010, with my former student, Professor Arjun Karki, as its driving force and first Vice Chancellor. So far, it functions as a medical school dedicated to training doctors who will work in Nepal and especially in remote areas. It has taken over the Lalitpur Nursing Campus and training of other health professionals is anticipated in the future.

I have been back on two visits to teach in the Medical School and give guest lectures to the weekly 'grand rounds' meeting. Arjun was keen that I should reprise the theme of 'Wonderland of Physiology' that I had used as a basis for several articles in the journal of the Institute of Medicine medical school when he was a student. I find that in spite of the passing of the years, my heart is still very much in Patan Hospital and it is delightful to find it involved in my other old love; educating medical students.

Was I a good Medical Director for Patan Hospital at that critical time? Of course, I can't really answer that, but I think the answer may be quite mixed. It was good that I had an excellent relation with Martyn Thomas during the completion of the building works, but I think I was less good in relations with those in authority. There was a time when certain authorities sought to replace me; I won't go into details. By that time I had got into the job and had been quite thrilled to see the way the hospital was developing, so I resisted this move. It came down to a consultation with the hospital staff and I'm glad to say they wanted me to stay. As the tipping point in my decision to take the job in the first place was a desire to support the staff, I found some justification in this result.

In 1985, though, came the realisation that we needed to return to UK for a period. Our parents were becoming frailer and our respective sisters and their families were carrying the load. Mary was by now in medical school in Cambridge and Jamie at the point of applying to a university, so they might well need some support too. We took the decision to leave the mission and Nepal, at least for some time, and this we did in 1986 after nearly four years at Patan.

Chapter 13.

Journeying to Woodstock. By Angela

Secondary education for the children posed a problem for expatriates working in Kathmandu. There was an excellent British Primary School , where our children had a good start up to the age of eleven, but the government at that time refused to let it expand and become a secondary school. There was an excellent American school, Lincoln, and Mary Joy had two valuable years there. However when it came to preparing for GCSE they told us that their curriculum would only cover twenty five per cent of the course. So we had to make the heart breaking decision about boarding school. Fortunately the mission was not able to pay for boarding school in UK. This would have meant long separations and living in very different worlds. By supplying teachers for two Christian boarding schools in India the mission was able to get discounts for the children.

We opted for Woodstock School in Mussoorie in NW India, which only took two days to reach from Kathmandu, whereas the alternative, Hebron, took five days to reach. There were two eighteen week terms. The winter holiday was two and a half months because it was too cold in Mussoorie in December January and February. There was a summer break in July for the monsoon. Parents were encouraged to rent a bungalow and take the children out of boarding especially for sports day and Gandhi's birthday, October 2nd, and May and June when the mothers were expected to help with all the end of term activities, the men joining them for some of the time. This meant that we would be together for almost half of the year which was not a bad compromise. However the journeys to Mussoorie from Kathmandu were hazardous.

A Look-see Visit

Mussoorie, Queen of the Hills, is a hill station very like Simla, the headquarters of the Raj in past times. It is approximately eight thousand feet above Dehra Dun. To this hill station still flock the inhabitants of Delhi to avoid the oppressive summer heat. In 1976 a friend and I made the journey from Kathmandu to the school with our children who were good friends and like cousins, to see what it was like. We borrowed four bedding rolls, one between two for the children. These are brightly coloured padded quilts which can be unrolled on a station platform and provide a reasonably comfortable bed to sleep on while waiting for a train. They can also turn into a mattress for the wooden slats that make up the sleeping berths on a train. No Indian would travel without one. We flew in a small Twin Otter to an air strip at Bhairawa. We then took a cycle rickshaw to the border. It took a while to get through the border checks even though in those days the English didn't need a visa. We took a train from Gorakhpur to Lucknow where we had to wait for the night train to Dehra Dun.

In Nepal, John's BMJ used to arrive addressed
Kathmandu
Nepal
India

This is the equivalent of sending a letter to
London
England
France

Nepal and India are perhaps more different than England and France. The mutual feelings of the countries towards one another are similar. The very first things that struck me in India were the vestiges of the Raj. Nepal was never under British rule so there are no vestiges of the Raj. The Indian trains are a legacy of the British. Unsurprisingly they were similar to our steam railways which are lovingly preserved in UK. The Indian trains were grimy from the smoke, very long, and jam packed, not only inside but on the roof as well, and incredibly cheap. Lucknow station itself looks as if Kings Cross or St Pancras had been transported. We went to the restaurant where the silverware equalled that of an officers' mess. My friend, a Tribhuwan University English tutor, asked and gestured "Tea for two and toast for six" It was far removed from a Nepali tea shop.

We spread our useful bedding rolls on the floor of the station rest room and waited for the night train to Dehra Dun. Our next challenge was to find the number of our compartment and berths. This information was posted on a notice board in Devanagri script. This was not a problem because Nepali is also written in Devanagri. Eventually we discovered our seat numbers under the name of "Mrs Mary". The train was late and there was a scuffle to board it. Our copious luggage was carried on the heads of tall porters, much taller than the Nepalese at that time, with very straight backs. We found that we had only been given three berths though we had paid for four. The ticket collector, perhaps because we were English, managed to persuade some people to move. So we spread out our bedding rolls on the berths, the children sharing with a head at each end, and settled down for the night. It wasn't long before passengers sat down on top of whoever was sleeping on the bottom bunks. Tales abounded of thieves who would steal your possessions during the night and even cut off watches from your wrist. At every station the cry of "*Garam chai*" would be heard. This was hot sweet tea, sold in little clay pots which would be then thrown out of the window. We finally arrived in Dehra Dun at half past nine the next morning, the train having made up time on the Deccan plain. The train would have left Calcutta forty eight hours earlier and generally arrived more or less on time at Dehra Dun. From Dehra Dun we took a taxi to Mussoorie. Dehra Dun is not much above sea level and Mussoorie is situated eight thousand feet above. The road zigzags up the mountain side. The skilled Sikh drivers would do the journey in forty minutes excluding vomit stops. We finally and thankfully arrived at our destination, which was Edge Hill Guest House.

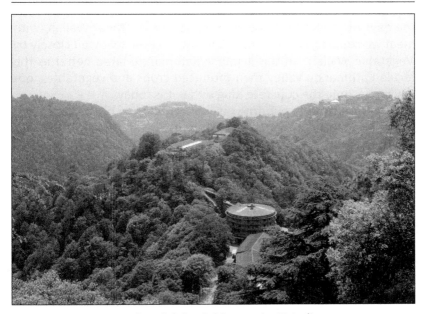

Woodstock School, Mussoorie, N. India

India seemed comparatively to have a wonderfully high standard of living. Nepal at that time was rated the second poorest country in the world. In Mussoorie, an English country parish church was another vestige of the Raj. In those days Nepalis were put in prison for changing their faith and Bibles had to be sold in an underhand way, in secret behind hidden shelves in certain bookshops. An open Christian bookshop in Mussoorie was heartening to see. There was very little to be had in Kathmandu, apart from rice, lentils, chickpeas and buffalo and goat meat. Mussoorie and Landour bazaar were full of interesting shops. The ultimate treat for us all, not just the children, was an ice cream at Quality's. At the top of the ridge in Sisters' Bazaar there was a clothes shop which did a roaring trade selling Punjabi outfits, (a short dress and baggy trousers), wrap around skirts, blouses, shirts, jewellery, sweets and cold drinks. We shopped rather too enthusiastically.

We were woken in the morning at the guest house with cries of "Bread Wallah" as a man with a basket full of loaves on his head arrived at the Guest House. This was followed shortly by "Cake Wallah" with a basket full of delicious cakes, the skill having been acquired during the days of the Raj. This was then followed by "Meat Wallah, with meat we could not have obtained in Kathmandu, followed closely by "Vegetable Wallah". In this instance Kathmandu fared better as the fertile Kathmandu valley then produced crops and vegetables, not having become the concrete jungle that it is today.

The return reverse journey went according to plan until we got to the Bhairawa airstrip. We were told that the plane was delayed. After buying some refreshments we had spent almost every rupee that we had. But as dark began to fall we realised that the plane was not going to come that day. We were going to have to spend the night in Bhairawa and we had practically no money. There were no landing lights in Kathmandu let alone Bhairawa airstrip. We all felt in our pockets for rupees and paisa that had got tucked away. Fortunately the children managed to discover quite a few paisa between them. This enabled us to rent a squalid room for the night. The plane arrived the next morning and took us safely back to Kathmandu. There had been no way of communicating with our husbands. However they had correctly assumed that the flight had not gone as the schedules were always erratic.

The four children had felt positive about going to Woodstock School. They had found the atmosphere very friendly. A school on an eight thousand foot ridge in the foothills of the Himalayas, looking north to the magnificent snowy peaks was not unlike Nepal. So the decision was made to go to Mussoorie the following year and eight years of regular faith-challenging travel from Kathmandu to Mussoorie ensued.

A variety of routes

The simplest way would have been to fly to Delhi and take the train from there but the cost of that flight was prohibitive. So initially we found that the best was to fly to Patna, take another flight to Lucknow and then the train to Dehra Dun and taxi to Mussoorie. It was important to book your train ticket in India fourteen days in advance. Inconveniently, the internet had not been invented then. We were helped by the good services of President Travel at the school and would have to send several letters to them as some usually got lost, asking them to organise tickets. The flight to Patna provided a wonderful post card view of Mount Everest. Once we had an after-noon and evening in Patna and went to the *Maidan* where numerous games of cricket were being played. A ball came our way and John bowled and by a fluke hit middle stump. The young Indian lads thought that he was Ian Botham. John often spoke with the men on these journeys and many expressed a wish that the British were still in India.

Although there was a group of us in the mission with children in Woodstock there were times when I had to make this journey alone. I was working at the mission Language and Orientation Centre at the time and my free times did not always coincide with those of anyone else. I have a vivid memory of trying to find my seat alone at Lucknow. I had worked out how to find my name quickly on the list. Everyone's age was noted so I just looked for the oldest person on the list and it was usually me –I must have been thirty nine at the time. However, finding the number on the list and translating that to the carriage and compartment was by no means easy. The trains were long, having vast numbers of carriages. The porters bearing your luggage on their heads were not able to help as they were often unable to read and write. I was very grateful to an educated young lad who saw my problem and offered to help me find my seat. This he did refusing to take any payment. There were special carriages for women which I tried to get when travelling alone. Jeremy Corbyn would have approved. During the summer months many Indians travel to a summer home in the hills. The women, dressed in beau-tiful coloured saris, were always very friendly and chatty. "We'll have a lovely journey together" they would say as we all packed in like sardines, insisting on sharing food and inviting me to their summer homes if they were going to be in Mussoorie or Landour.

Times and air routes change and by and by Indian Airlines stopped the flight from Patna to Lucknow so we had to find other ways of accomplishing the two day journey. About that time Britain insisted on Indians getting a visa when they came to Britain and so India nat-urally insisted that the British needed a visa for India. We could go on a tourist visa but the children needed a student visa and could not enter on a tourist visa and then change it. This was readily given but extremely time consuming to obtain. So there were added difficulties.

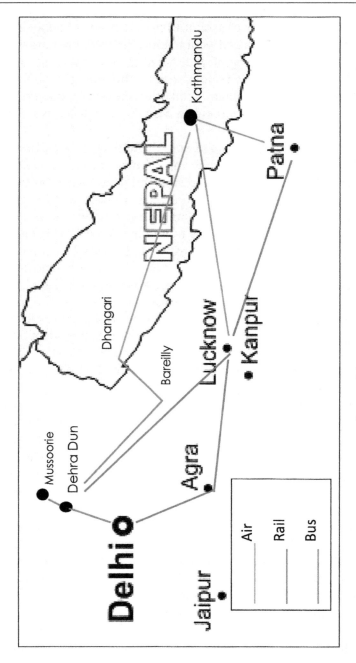

Some of the routes to Mussoorie.

We must have tried every conceivable route. Sometimes we bussed back from Dehra Dun to Delhi in part joining the Grand Trunk Road, so vividly described in Rudyard Kipling's Kim, still with its bullock carts, wayside shrines and numerous tea stalls. Our half way stop was at a Deer Park with a more hygienic restaurant selling drinks and samosas, welcome in temperatures of over forty centigrade. From Delhi on one luxurious occasion we travelled in an air conditioned coach with upright seats and no one sitting on top of us.

One adventurous journey, which as far as I know John and I were the only parents to try out, was via Dhanghadi, an airstrip in the far West of Nepal. We had asked our paediatrician to ask her parents who lived in Barreilly, to get us train tickets from Bareilly to Dehra Dun. We intended to fly to Dhanghadi, take a rickshaw to the border, a bus through bandit country to Barreilly and from there to take the train to Dehra Dun. Our Nepali friends were concerned about us travelling through bandit country. We were instructed if we were held up by Indian "highwaymen" to surrender everything we had rather than lose our lives. The flight was late. It was also much further to travel from the airstrip to the border than it appeared on the map. At the border we got on a bus guarded by an elderly soldier with an elderly gun who stood looking out at the front. Fortunately we did not encounter any bandits. Inevitably by the time we reached Barreilly the train had long since come and gone. So we found a ramshackle night bus and endured an uncomfortable journey to Dehra Dun. The taxi from Dehra Dun seemed very luxurious. However we had just had one sleepless night. I found it difficult to cope with two sleepless nights as happened on an occasion when we went via Varanasi, although I can't remember exactly what went wrong. I think it had something to do with riots at the time.

Meanwhile our children usually flew to Delhi where they were met by members of school staff and taken with a school party to Woodstock. This meant that Mary Joy, aged thirteen and Jamie aged eleven had to travel from Kathmandu to Delhi on their own. When we asked if they could have special help from the airhostess we were told that Mary Joy at thirteen was classified as an adult and Jamie aged eleven was therefore travelling with an adult. On one occasion we said Goodbye to them at the airport, saw them go through the barrier and assumed that they were on their way to Delhi. Later that day we got a phone call from the nearby Narayani Hotel. The flight had been cancelled and Indian Airlines were putting them up at the Narayani hotel. "Would you like to come home?" we asked. They would not. They were having a great time going up and down in the lift, a novelty for them. The Nepali hotel staff had no problem with this; the guests may have been less amused. We joined our children for dinner, choosing the least expensive item on the menu, whereas with their Indian Airlines voucher they chose the most expensive.

There is no other carrot that would have persuaded me to undertake these journeys, especially on my own, if it had not been to spend time with our children. A friend of mine once said "It is important for our children to go to a school that they can love". I think that our children did go to a school that they could love: and I suspect that they were among the last British mission children to be educated in India.

John's note.

I want to include a word or two about my wife, Angela. As I have explained, she was an Oxford graduate, a talented teacher and even a talented actress who had played parts on BBC radio. Yet she chose to devote herself to the children for the first few years and then took on all the administration of getting them to boarding school in India and supporting them there. This involved getting visas, air tickets and all the necessary clothes and kit for the term. She did more of the visiting than I did and stayed longer, though sometimes we went together and on occasions I had mission meetings in Delhi which enabled me to make a side trip to the school. The expression 'holding the family together' comes to mind, and Angela was the one who did it.

Sending children away to school is inevitably an emotional event, but she coped with it better than I had expected. She explained that, like the White Queen in Alice through the Looking Glass, she did her crying before the event.

As well as this, she was the one who took responsibility for keeping in touch with our supporters at home and did a lot of the tedious jobs like dealing with the Nepal Tax Office.

There was a lot of pressure on her to take on jobs within the mission, but only after the kids were in Boarding School did she agree to any of the suggestions. She did some part time French teaching at the British Primary School, even while the kids were attending it, and began giving some English classes at the Shanta Bhawan Nursing School. (Somewhat to my annoyance, the students called her 'Angela Miss'!) Later, she took on the responsibility of administering the Mission's Orientation Programme for new arrivals and did so with great energy and efficiency.

In later years, she devoted herself largely to teaching English at the nursing school, now renamed the Lalitpur Nursing Campus. For this she took a qualification in Teaching English as a Foreign Language (TEFL). Some of the students she taught went on to become 'Campus Chiefs' in other schools and she was frequently greeted in the street by former pupils.

Chapter 14.

Customs, Culture and Religion

Namaste! This is the usual Nepali (and Indian) greeting. It is derived from the Sanskrit, *'namah'* and *'te'*, and its meaning is something like "I bow to the god in you". I suspect that most Nepalese don't actually think of this as they use the salutation, any more than English speakers think "God be with you" when they say "Goodbye", but it is an indicator of a major gap in understanding between Christians and Hindus when talking about religion.

A different World View

You see, Christians think of God as being entirely separate from humans and the rest of his creation, whereas, at least on a philosophical level, both Hindus and Buddhists believe in the 'oneness' of the world. For them meditation is a means of realising that we are part of god and god is part of us, and becoming at one with the infinite. Buddhists would see this realisation, at its fullest, leading them out of the cycle of re-incarnation and into nirvana. For some Hindus, at least, this is possible, but only through many lifetimes of re-incarnation; 'karma' or deeds, actions, leading to a better re-incarnation each time. It is no wonder that we find ourselves talking at cross purposes.

Coming from a country that is nominally Christian, at least, I found it hard to walk among the crowds in *Naya Sadak* (New Road) in Kathmandu and think that not one of those hundreds of people passing me or in the shops was also a Christian. I felt like an alien; and so I was! Our entire world view was different.

Of course, for many Hindus and Buddhists their religion is not of the philosophical kind. The expression of their belief lies in the worship of many gods. It is said that there are 330 million gods in Hinduism, though the Rig Veda lists only 33 and some would argue that they are all manifestations of the supreme god, *Param Ishwar*. Nepali Christians have adopted the name '*Parmeshwar*' to represent God, but this has the potential for misunderstanding.

Popular religion in Nepal, therefore, consists of household and temple worship of gods, and festivals dedicated to them. The King of Nepal was regarded as the manifestation of a god and the 'living goddesses' of Kathmandu, Patan and elsewhere are also worshipped. They are generally chosen as small girls and fulfil their roles as objects of worship until the time when they first shed blood.

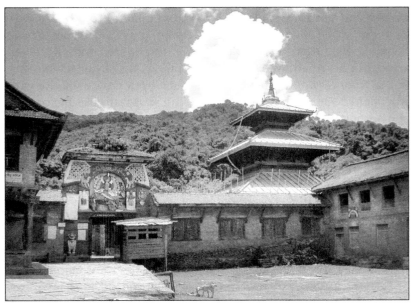

Typical Hindu Temple

Apart from the King and the living goddesses, the gods are mostly represented by idols. These can be elaborate statues with the particular characteristics of the god they represent, or, alternatively, rough images or even stones. Close to where we lived, there was a large stone embedded in the tarmac of a road and people were to be seen offering it flowers, fruit and worship. This stone had traditionally been worshipped as a god and so the road had simply been built around it.

Idols can be paraded around the streets in particular festivals and even for several weeks at a time as in the annual Rato Macchendranath festival in Patan. Macchendranath is installed in a traditional chariot with a high spire-like structure and this chariot is prone to overturning and fouling telephone and electricity wires, as well as blocking roads.

Gods can also be represented by animals. The cow is an obvious example. Cows and bulls wander freely among the traffic in Kathmandu and woe betide anyone who injures one. An American friend working in a rural mission hospital was proud of his vegetable garden and used his khukri (a large curved knife) to attack a wandering cow that fed on it. This led to a major upheaval; he could have been expelled from the district or from the entire country or even killed, but negotiations eventually resulted in his paying a large fine. At the *Tihar (Diwali)* festival, not only cows, but crows and dogs are worshipped. On other occasions, even cars, buses, trucks, helicopters and aeroplanes are worshipped as well.

Karma

The Hindu concept of *'Karma'* can also lead to misunderstanding. It should not be over-simplified, but it contains the idea that doing good deeds can lead to a better re-incarnation. I have speculated that this is one reason why there is no traditional word for "thank you" in Nepali (though *'dhanyabad'* has been adopted from Sanskrit). Traditionally, if you buy something in a shop, the transaction simply ends with "Take the goods" and "Take the money". Perhaps this is because the deed is seen as its own reward in terms of karma; both sides benefit and gratitude is irrelevant.

I had an interesting experience with this mind set. I was at a conference on TB in Biratnagar, a town in the east of the country and near the southern border. The subject of discussion was the use of volunteers in TB control. One Nepali doctor said: "It's no use depending on people to do something for nothing. Look at the Christian missionaries." He continued, "They only do their good works so that they can earn their seats in heaven!" As I was the only missionary present, I thought I ought to reply and explained that I don't have to earn my 'seat' in heaven; it's something the Lord Jesus earned for me on the Cross. Not wanting to get too heavy, I said that in fact I was more certain of my 'seat' in heaven than I was of my seat on the flight to Kathmandu that evening. As it turned out, the flight was cancelled and I spent the evening talking about my seat on the flight and my seat in heaven! As I said, clear communication is difficult when you have such different world views.

Church, Persecution and Mission

When we first arrived in 1969, we found Nepal to be fiercely proud of having never been a colony of Britain or any other country, and also of being the only Hindu Kingdom in the world. It was illegal under national law, the *'mulki ain'*, to change one's religion, which meant in effect to be anything other than a Hindu. This needs a bit of clarifying, as Buddhism was officially seen as a form of Hinduism, which certainly applies to much of Nepalese Buddhism, but not necessarily to those related to Tibetan, tantric or lamaistic Buddhism. The upshot of this was that after Christianity first entered Nepal in the modern era in the early 1950s, new Christians were very often put into prison for their faith as they had broken the law. Anyone who was held responsible for their conversion was also liable to be imprisoned. Baptism was seen as the point of conversion and pastors preparing people seeking baptism asked them to affirm that they were prepared to go to prison for the step they were about to take. When Nepali pastors administered baptism they were also at risk of imprisonment.

From the point of view of officialdom, this was almost certainly counter-productive. Under this kind of persecution, the faith of the growing church became strong and 'rice Christians' were unknown. From the material point of view, there was nothing to be gained by becoming a Christian, and much to lose. Many did go to prison, and

145

other prisoners became Christian. We knew at least one Christian married couple who had met each other in prison.

This official persecution gradually weakened until Nepal was declared a secular state in 2006 and the claim to be the world's only Hindu Kingdom ceased to have any meaning with the overthrow of the monarchy in 2007.

From the point of view of Christian missions, we in UMN were under an agreement with the government not to 'proselytise'. It was difficult to know what this meant exactly, but behind it seemed to be the historical invasion of India by Muslims and the policy of 'Islam or the Sword'. We were certainly not interested in that sort of evangelism! In practice, we felt that we could join Nepali churches, but not take leadership positions. We could speak in church if asked, but not preach at any public meetings. At Shanta Bhawan, we could hold services on Sunday, but in the Library, not in the wards, so that patients would feel free to attend but not under any compulsion. We could give people Bibles and other Christian books if they were willing to accept them, but there should be no element of coercion. On the whole, government seemed to accept these practices on the part of missionaries, and I do not recall any confrontation concerning our mission.

Nepalese Christians were often persecuted by their families and neighbours. I stayed in a home in a remote village where my Christian hosts were denied permission to take water from the village well, and this was quite a common situation. Parents in some cases refused to acknowledge sons and daughters who had become Christian. I know of one mother who committed suicide, allegedly because of her son's conversion.

Family is definitely important to Hindus! I used to have long talks with an intellectual (PhD) who is convinced of the rightness of the Gospel but would not take the step of alienating his parents. Added to the common view that 'all ways lead to god' in his background, this has led him to be a long term fence-sitter and this is an uncomfortable position in every sense.

Growth of the Church

It is hard to deny that the rapid growth of the Nepali church was in part due to two influences; the **effect of persecution** and the complete **absence of any foreign leadership** in the churches.

When we first arrived, there were only about 500 Christians in Nepal, including expatriates. Now there are certainly well over a million and churches are to be found in cities, towns and villages all over the country, possibly 40 or more in the Kathmandu Valley. Christmas Day is recognised as a holiday, though not as a government holiday. [*Angela says:* There are also now more than 30 Nepali Christian fellowships in UK, as well as some in Germany, Portugal and the Netherlands and elsewhere.]

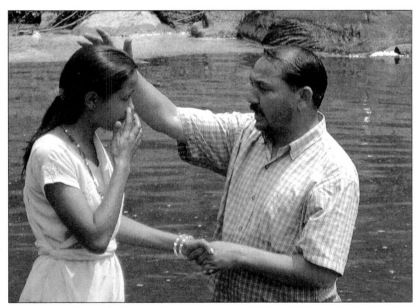

Christian Baptism. Photo: Dr Alan Young

Part of the background to all this is the fact that Hinduism is not a missionary religion. Someone born into a Hindu family is by definition a Hindu and is unalterably a member of the caste of his family. So it is not possible to become a Hindu in the way that one can become a Christian. (There are a few exceptions, for example in the Hare Krishna movement and other guru sects.)

Various customs cause misunderstanding. Hindu brides wear red and are puzzled that Christians wear white, which for them is the colour of death. Hindus marry only on 'auspicious' days according to the astrological calendar. I recall one hippie couple who got married and arranged everything according to the Hindu rites, except, as one Nepali commented bitingly "They got married on a day when only dogs marry!" High caste Hindu males shave their heads as a sign of bereavement and this was a cause of tension when King Birendra was killed. [See Chapter 18.] Some Christians shaved their heads in mourning, but their pastors saw it as slipping back into Hindu ways.

On various ceremonial occasions, Christians are offered *'tika'*, a red mark on the forehead, quite possibly as a sign of friendship, but it can also represent an offering made to an idol, so Christians are unwilling to accept it.

Hindus do not eat beef out of their veneration for the cow, Which according to some versions, uses its horns to open the door to the next re-incarnation. This is understandable, but a puzzling common misconception about Christians is that they are positively obliged to eat beef as part of their religion!

Caste

I'm going to write a bit about caste, though it is a hard concept for non-Hindus to understand and I admit to the possibility of getting it wrong. I have referred to the way food has to be cooked by the 'right' caste; otherwise it is defiled and uneatable, at least to the higher castes. The *Brahmins* are traditionally priests, scholars and teachers, though they are commonly found in other occupations. The Chettris (or *Kshattriyas*) are the warrior caste, though they are now more often to be found in other jobs. The *Vaishyas* are shopkeepers, farmers and some artisans and many of the tribes fit into this caste, including many of those recruited into the British Army as 'Gurkhas'. The *Sudras* are labourers and people providing services, such as tailors and musicians. Other occupational groups, though, are considered untouchable or *dalit*, such as the metal workers (*kami*), leather workers (*sarki*), laundrymen (*dhobi*) and bonded labourers. The large Newar tribe has its own caste system.

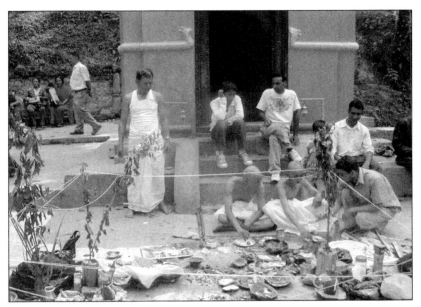

Sacred Thread Ceremony for High Caste Hindu Boys.

Discrimination against untouchables has been illegal for many years in Nepal, but of course it continues. We had a very low caste porter on one trek and he had very poor self-esteem. This meant that he could not carry out usual porter's tasks such as buying food or negotiating an arrangement for us to sleep on the veranda of a village house. The kids named him 'Puddleglum' for his habitual pessimism about the way he expected to be treated.

As I have described, our first house was at the end of a path used by the locals as a public toilet. (This was the 'Primrose Path' to adults and 'Ooey Alley' to the kids.) Hearing about this, our supporting church, (the excellent St James the Less in Bethnal Green, London) was alarmed and concerned enough to raise some money for the construction of a small, rough, public toilet beside the path. The hospital maintenance department built this structure and the local people were asked to ensure that it was kept clean. Sadly, the response was "Our caste doesn't clean toilets!" This was regrettable but predictable and the whole project turned into a bit of a flop, though some people did use it. [*Jamie says:* This was an area to avoid if you were wearing flip flops–really!!]

The Gurkhas are generally not particularly caste-conscious. However a large number of them retired from the service at about the time of Hong Kong's reversion to China and the building of a new airport to the north of Lantau Island. This required a bridge link of 2 ½ miles and welders were required in large numbers. Initially the Gurkhas turned up their noses at this employment as '*kami*'s work', but their attitude changed when the pay scales for welders were revealed as quite generous!

I had thought to call this chapter "Clash of Cultures", which seemed suitably dramatic and alliterative. But, thinking about it, there need not be a clash. It just needs time and flexibility to under-stand other peoples' world view, traditions and customs and to learn to accept them. I think of so many Nepali friends who are so different from me and yet we relate so well. There is a lesson for newcomers, one that I always pass on to medical students going to Nepal for their electives, for example; keep your ears and eyes open and your mouth shut until you have really understood the reasons for the way things are.

Chapter 15.

The British Army and the Gurkhas

As I have said at the end of Chapter 12, we needed some time in UK. I am not going to recount this in detail, but will describe our on-going connections with Nepal and the Gurkhas.

The Brigade of Gurkhas consists of British officers and Nepalese officers and soldiers recruited from Nepal. In 2015, the Brigade celebrated the 200th anniversary of its foundation, which was remarkable considering that in 1815 Nepal and the British East India Company were at war with each other! (Some Nepalese had been recruited earlier.)

How did I come to be an Army Physician? [*Angela says:* There were various possibilities of jobs at the time. I thought the army was so unlikely that I never gave it any thought.] Well, it all began when I was invited to give a short lecture at a medical seminar to celebrate the 25th anniversary of the British Military Hospital in Dharan in Eastern Nepal. I was asked to speak about my experience with the first medical school. At the time, the Commanding Officer was Lt Col Guy Ratcliffe, who became a good friend and colleague later. During the visit, in which I stayed with Guy and Maggi, he said he was expecting a visit from some military medical 'brass' from UK and would like to bring them to see Patan Hospital. So a few weeks later I was standing with a small group on the roof of the hospital pointing out the various Himalayan peaks, when the Brigadier asked me how long I was expecting to stay in Nepal. Learning that I was planning to leave the following year, he followed with asking what I intended to do. I had a few ideas, but nothing certain, so he said "Why don't you join the Royal Army Medical Corps?"

To cut a long story short, that is what I did. I attended a Commissioning Board at Millbank, where I was asked whether, as a Christian missionary, I would have any difficulty about carrying a weapon in order to protect myself and my patients. I replied, perhaps a bit impertinently, that if the world was as God made it, we would have no need of armies and no need of doctors! As it is, unfortunately, we need both and, yes, I would carry a weapon if required. (Mercifully, I never was!)

One of Jamie's best lines was delivered when I told him I was going to join the Army. Leaning over from his 6'3" or so; "Dad, I think the army will make a man of you!"

Though I expected this phase to last 3-4 years, it actually lasted for over thirteen. In brief, I did four months' training, including a month at Sandhurst, then postings at Military Hospitals in Woolwich and Catterick (twice), the RAF hospital in Akrotiri in Cyprus and ended up as Head of Postgraduate Medical Education for the three Services at the Royal Defence Medical College, then in Gosport, a very Naval town. I also served in a Field Hospital in the First Gulf War in 1991, of which more later.

Sandhurst and the Gurkhas.

I was part of a course for doctors, dentists, chaplains and other professional types joining the army as officers. The Demonstration Company consists of Gurkhas who are, of course, extremely well trained and experienced soldiers. As well as demonstrating certain skills, they acted as the enemy in our simulated attacks. As the incompetent horde of doctors etc. came over the hill and towards their trenches, they were trained to fall over dead with barely a struggle. However, in my case, I could flop down under the cover of their trench and have a good natter with them in Nepali, which surprised them, but their eyes lit up at this novelty.

The First Gulf War and the Gurkhas

At the end of 1990 I found I was to be posted to 22 Field Hospital in Saudi Arabia in support of the Allied Desert Shield operation, which became Operation Desert Storm with the beginning of the Gulf War on 17 January 1991. After some training for the desert, some of which took place hilariously on the snow-covered Feldom Ranges, we left for Al Jubail in early January. We were camped on a huge car park in this town on the east coast of Saudi Arabia for more training, especially in Nuclear Biological and Chemical (NBC) warfare defence as it was known that Saddam Hussein had chemical and possibly biological weapons in his armoury.

It turned out that one of the NBC instructors was a Gurkha sergeant and I got to know him quite well. He told me that there were Gurkhas at another camp nearby and we went together for a fine *daal-bhat* meal with them. There was a squadron of Gurkha Transport and the Gurkha band. When I recalled this sergeant, I could not remember his name, but, strangely, I met him again in Yorkshire. By this time, he had retired with the most senior commissioned rank of Gurkha Major and had been employed for some years as Operations Manager at Harewood House, a stately home north of Leeds. So now I know him as the much-respected Laxmi Bantawa and I arranged for him to make a presentation on life as a Gurkha in Richmond. We have got to know his wife and 3 daughters and twice enjoyed *daal-bhat* with them in their cottage in the grounds of Harewood House.

Back to the Gulf; when we went forward to our tent hospital in the desert, I found to my delight that half of the Gurkha transport squadron and half of the band was part of our Unit. The traditional wartime role of bandsmen in the army is casualty recovery, so they were able to work together with the other Gurkhas to form an Ambulance Squadron.

One evening they were telling me that, though they were trained in First Aid and casualty recovery, they had never actually inserted a cannula (a thick needle} into the vein of a real person for the purpose of giving fluids or blood. So I spent the rest of the evening allowing them to put drips into my arms and instructing them in the technique. This was probably foolish, as my arms were distinctly sore next day and they never had to do it for real.

In the end, we took very few Allied casualties and the main value of our presence proved to be the care of Iraqi prisoners of war. Contrary to their initial apprehensions, they were treated very well.

The nearest threat to our own safety was when a Scud missile thumped into the desert a few miles away. We all scrambled into our NBC suits, but it turned out not to have a biological or chemical payload.

The ground war, which had started on the 24th February, ended on the 3rd of March. Both before and after the hostilities, I was involved in organising concerts for the unit and was asked to arrange some Gurkha items. These were a great success, though the fierce-looking Khukri Dance had the front row spectators leaning backwards in fear of the flashing blades. There was a hilarious Tharu dance miming hunting in the jungle, hunger and the production of two eggs from within a skimpy loin cloth. The bandsmen did some musical items which were excellent considering they had none of their proper instruments available. No problem! They improvised using water bottles tuned by adding different amounts of water and the drums from the empty spindles of wiring supplies. They asked me to explain to the audience a traditional G*urkha song, the* Dehra Dune Git. This was sung in Dehra Dun, which had been the site of the Gurkha Depot in British India. The song commemorated the colleagues who had fallen in the Mesopotamia Campaign. This was clearly relevant as the Allies were expecting to advance into Iraq. (In the end, we did not need to follow the tanks as they met little resistance and suffered few casualties.)

I ended my involvement in the Gulf War rather ignominiously. In short, I fell into the burning pit with all the other rubbish! This was the day before we were due to leave and my feet were too damaged for me to wear my boots. So I had to be taken to 33 Field Hospital, which was still just functional, to be evacuated by helicopter. There I met with more Gurkhas and had interesting chats. One was a Christian, which was quite unusual in those days. They told me that they had really done nothing much during the war and would be ashamed to be awarded medals. They had in mind the tribulations of their predecessors fighting in Burma, Malaya and other conflicts, including Mesopotamia, which was where the Gulf War *dushman* (enemy) had come from. In the end, like me, they got medals from MoD and from the Saudi and Kuwaiti governments. This was certainly overkill, but the last two were only to be worn in the presence of Royalty or Ambassadors of these respective countries.

Nepal with the Army

As a hospital physician, I could not be appointed Medical Officer to a Gurkha unit as that was a job for a GP. Because of my Nepali language and Nepal experience, though, I was sent for short attachments to Nepal. The first of these was to replace the physician at the BMH Dharan who was returning to UK for his consultant appointment Board (ASCAB). Later visits were for Gurkha recruiting medicals and for medical treks to Area Welfare Centres under the auspices of the Gurkha Welfare Trust. On average, I think I went about every two years.

The recruiting process was interesting. For one thing, my first partner as Medical Officer was a Royal Navy Radiologist; probably the first naval officer to be sent on duty to this landlocked country. He was gob-smacked by what he saw and not best pleased when I took him on an early morning climb to a high viewpoint of Sarangkot in celebration of my 50th birthday!

It was extraordinary to find that none of the young candidates had any sign of dental caries; a tribute to their traditional, virtually sugar-free diet. We went to observe the test of fitness and stamina. The recruits each filled a *dhoko* (the traditional carrying basket with a *namlo* or headband), with 25 kg of rocks from the river bed and then, on command, raced to the top of a ridge some 3000 feet above them carrying this load. Though I was quite fit, I knew that I could not have carried that load to the top without rest stops, let alone run the whole way with it as most of them were able to do.

A longer posting in Nepal came in 1995-6. The impending handover of Hong Kong from Britain to China in 1997 was to have major effects on the Gurkhas, not least on their health care. Until that time, any long term health problem that needed special care involving Gurkha soldiers or their dependents would result in a posting to Hong Kong and managed in the British Military Hospital there or in local civilian facilities. Clearly things would have to change and it was my job to make the necessary arrangements for their care in Nepal itself.

So I was sent on a Temporary Manning Attachment to the British Gurkhas Kathmandu and the Gurkha Welfare Trust. This lasted about a year and a quarter and Angela and I were accommodated in a magnificent large house, quite different from the days with the mission. We were expected to employ five servants. However, we kept it to three. First our old friend Sita; second, an excellent, though somewhat surly, cook called Sunder and lastly a live-in *'chowkidar'* (gatekeeper) cum gardener, Bimal. The house had a generator, water delivered by tanker, water-purifying gadgets and all sorts of luxuries that we had never known.

There were three main parts to my task. First, assisted by a SSAFA sister, I was to search for suitable facilities in Nepal for all of the long term sick, including some extremely disabled children and several organ transplant cases. Second, I was to upgrade the medical rooms in the Area Welfare Centres, (AWCs), training the medics and appointing new ones when necessary. Lastly, I was to do this without costing anyone any money! It was a typical government 'cost-neutral' exercise and I thought it might be doomed to failure.

Fortunately, I discovered that the medical rooms were being ripped off by local contractors in the annual medical supplies purchase. This allowed me to make alternative arrangements, using my contacts in the mission, to get better, more reliable and cheaper medicines. This gave a bit more latitude for expenditure.

I was able to draw up a large database of people with chronic health problems and their requirements. Using this I was gradually able to make arrangements and work out possible costs.

One illustrative problem was the number of people who had undergone kidney or liver transplant operations in other countries. More expertise had developed in Nepal by this time, but the problem was expense. The drugs used to prevent rejection of the transplanted organ have to be taken for life and are very expensive. I wonder what those who had performed these operations had thought would happen in the long run. The British Government has been generous to Gurkhas over the years, but there are limits and I was told to apply them. In the end, I was able to reach a reasonable solution under which they would get their drugs free from GWT and be supervised by Nepalese renal physicians.

Part of the job involved visiting Hong Kong, Singapore and Brunei. Angela was able to join me in these places as well as on one trip to the Area Welfare Centres in Darjeeling and Kalimpong in India. We certainly enjoyed these trips and I think they were a little more than 'jollies' because I learnt quite a lot and made good contacts.

Other visits were to most of the AWCs within Nepal. The ones in the East of the country were mostly only accessible by foot. You can imagine that I was not unduly chagrined to find that I was to be paid for walking through some of my favourite mountain countryside and staying with the retired Gurkhas who manned these AWCs.

As an officer, I was expected to trek with four porters and an interpreter/ guide. I managed to talk my way out of the interpreter as I could understand and speak for myself, and I managed to get away with only 3 porters, which is still quite an establishment for one man who was actually quite capable of wandering through the hills on his own. Again, it was the height of luxury. On top of the basket of one of the porters rode a folding chair for the 'Doctor Saheb'. This was unshipped and set up with ceremony at any stopping place, lest he should sully his bum sitting on a rock! They also carried a flask with tea or coffee for me and performed the usual trekking duties of making camp, providing hot water and cooking meals. After my many treks with Saila, I was accustomed to helping find firewood and carry water (unskilled tasks within my ability), but this I was not allowed to do.

At the AWCs, the Area Welfare Officers and their assistants were a delight. They were full of stories of their lives in the Service and of the various people we knew in common. There were supplies of '*tongba*' around the table; a millet-based alcoholic drink served with hot water in traditional pots in the East of Nepal. Sometimes there was *rakshi*, which can be extremely potent, and bottled beer.

In the morning, there was an early rise, a ritual cleaning up of the Centre, some tea and maybe chapattis and time for work. I would check the equipment and drug inventory with the 'medic', usually a Health Assistant, and examine the patient records. (I had devised a new, systematic form that encouraged logical thinking and recording in questioning, examining, reaching a diagnosis and treating each patient. Previously notes of the 'fever–aspirin' type had been the norm.) Then I would see any patients that came for treatment, teaching the health assistant as I went along. This could take some time, but would be interrupted by *'daal bhat'*, the standard mid-morning meal.

Generally in the middle of the day it was time to set out for the next AWC, but not without ceremony! I would usually be presented with a *'mala'*, a flower garland that I had to wear as I set out. At first, it was hard to know just what to do with it, but I learned that it was acceptable to walk a mile or two and then hang it respectfully on a suitable branch. At times, I was given other gifts, such as a ceremonial *khukri*, the curved knife used as a weapon by the Gurkhas and a domestic implement all over Nepal. I'm afraid my collection of *khukris* grew over large!

Though I was always welcome at the AWCs, there was a certain amount of resentment against me in the chronically-sick section of the Gurkha community. I felt a bit like a referee awarding a penalty against the home side. Many had been receiving Rolls-Royce treatment in Hong Kong and I was the one arranging for them to have what they perceived as very inferior care in Nepal instead. "It's just my job!" would not really hack it.

Overall, we have some happy memories of this interlude, including playing tennis and basketball with the Gurkhas, running an early-morning downhill half marathon and some memorable social occasions. [*Angela says* (being better at priorities): We were also able to link up with Nepali Christian and missionary friends.]

Basketball was particularly interesting. The Nepalese generally lack the height necessary for excellence at the game, but make up for it by speed and determination. The determination part of it conflicts with the conception found in most other parts of the world that basketball is not a contact sport. Mary came on a holiday and got involved in a basketball game for women in front of most of the Camp. I think that she and a British officer's wife were the only ones who had actually played the game before and both were quite good. The match was hilariously entertaining for players and spectators.

I retired from the Army in 2000 after something over 13 years of service and we returned (this time without kids) to five more years of service with the mission in Nepal. This is an odd story, I know; what I call my mission-military sandwich of a life.

Chapter 16.

Return to Nepal.

W hen we decided to return to UK in 1986, I thought it would only be a matter of three years or so before we returned to the mission. In the end, though, we did not go back until the New Millennium, April 2000. If I had had my choice, I would have returned to clinical work at Patan Hospital, or perhaps even as Medical Director. But I had correspondence with David Weakliam, an Irishman I came to respect for his work as Health Services Secretary for United Mission to Nepal as well as a good tennis opponent. David wanted me to become Director of the Sakriya Unit, which was UMN's response to the HIV/AIDS epidemic in the country. I knew very little about it, but I set out on yet another new career in HIV and community health.

I was able to make use of some of my Army resettlement time ('gardening leave') to study the subject and to spend time in the old Mildmay Mission Hospital in Bethnal Green, London which had become an AIDS hospice. This was a considerable eye opener and the learning curve was a steep one. Among other things, I was criticised for bowling into the room of a patient and taking charge in the way to which I was accustomed as a Consultant Physician. It seems I was expected to ask permission before even going into the room! After all, it was the only home the patient had. All very instructive, not to mention humiliating! As David had asked me also to be involved with the Nepal Government TB Control Centre, I also took the opportunity of attending a TB conference in Edinburgh in which the dynamic head of the centre, Dr Bam, was also taking part.

HIV in Nepal

HIV was first detected in Nepal in 1988, some 17 years after a strange disease was recognised in gay men in California. When it first appeared in Nepal, I was serving in an Army Hospital in Woolwich and seeing the condition for the first time myself. In fact, I found myself under surveillance for the disease! I had been investigating a soldier of African origin for a tropical disease and part of this involved taking skin snips to look for parasites. It was a bloody procedure and I was certainly exposed to a quantity of his blood! A day or two later suspicions hardened and were proved; he had AIDS! So I had a series of blood tests over the next few months to see if I had 'seroconverted'. Thankfully, I hadn't.

Briefly, though Nepal did not have anything like the heavy epidemic of HIV found in many African countries, the condition was being identified with increasing frequency. There were a number of sociological practices that led to this. One was migrant labour in India. Men would leave their wives behind, work in Indian towns in hotels or restaurants and console themselves with prostitutes (more properly known as Commercial Sex Workers, CSWs, in the jargon). This resulted in their bringing the infection home to be shared with their unfortunate wives. A second factor was the trafficking of Nepali girls to work in India as CSWs, mostly, but not always, against their will. They would be 'retired' to Nepal. A third and large factor was the increasing number of Injecting Drug Users in Nepal, some of whom were CSWs. One could recognise overlapping networks of these groups. There were also men who have sex with men (MSMs), though they were very much underground in those days.

Sakriya Unit

'*Sakriya*' means active or dynamic. The unit was very small and we soon had to find bigger premises and recruit more staff. It had been set up by the excellent Sally Smith, who later went on to work for WHO. The main function at the time was 'Awareness Raising' and

I had to start learning the current jargon in community health and management. People were delegated by UMN projects and many other organisations to come to us for a training course in HIV and how to pass on knowledge of the risks to members of their own work places and communities. This was led by Bishnu Ghimire who is a very energetic and committed worker.

In addition, we moved into the training of HIV/AIDS counsellors and produced a well-received training manual in Nepali.

I will not go into greater detail about the HIV/AIDS work here, but have reproduced as Appendix V an article which I wrote at a time when I was actively involved in the struggle to contain AIDS.

In 2003, I recommended to UMN that Sakriya Unit was ready to become an independent Nepali Non-Government Organisation (NGO) and I was able to go on home assignment, leaving it in the safe hands of Bishnu as the Director. It was renamed Sakriya Sewa Samaj, meaning roughly Active Service Society, and it has an expanding role in several of the more severely affected districts.

Christians and HIV

Christians have been involved extensively in the response to the HIV/AIDS epidemic, for example at the Mildmay Mission Hospital in London and the Sakriya Unit in Nepal. However, there is a risk that our attitude may be misunderstood. As do any medical workers, we treat all patients equally without any discrimination and without apportioning blame. But, it may be objected, some of the lifestyle practices that lead to HIV infection must surely be abhorrent to Christians, so how can they maintain non-discriminatory standards? Christian teaching certainly warns against sexual promiscuity, sex outside of marriage and homosexual practices, in contrast to the liberal spirit of the current age which holds them to be normal.

But consider the woman whose husband brings back HIV infection from India or their baby born later. Their lifestyle has not contributed to their resulting infection and illness. In the same way, many of the girls forced into sex work had no choice in the matter. It is wrong to judge others, as well, partly because it is impossible to know their full story, partly because it is not at all helpful in treating or counselling them, but mainly because Christians believe God is the ultimate judge and judgements should be left to him.

Anger, on the other hand, is not forbidden to Christians, especially when confronted with injustice and exploitation. I believe that most people with any kind of faith, or none, share our anger against those who traffic girls for sex and peddle drugs of addiction. A very good Nepali organisation is active in rescuing girls who have been forced into sex work and in exposing those who make a profit from ruining their lives.

Hospitals again

During my time at Sakriya, David Weakliam asked me if I would also take on the role of Deputy Health Services Director for Hospitals. There was a sense that the government would like the two remaining UMN mission hospitals to pass into Nepali hands, though the government did not seem to want to take them under its own responsibility as the challenge of funding and staffing them would have been too great. At the same time, the mission itself was under increasing financial pressures and a sense that the time to hand over the hospitals had come.

My task was to negotiate solutions that would preserve the integrity of the two hospitals, at Tansen and Okhaldhunga and satisfy both the government and the mission Board. The likely options were to hand the hospitals to either Christian NGOs or local hospital boards. To cut a long story short, neither option proved workable. I left the position in 2003 to go on home leave having not achieved the object. I should say that none of my successors achieved it either and the two hospitals are still being run by the mission some 12 years later. They are also doing a very good job; Tansen received a 'Best Hospital' award recently and Okhaldhunga is expanding with an extensive building programme.

Back to Medical Education

After our return from UK in 2003, it was all change professionally again. Sakriya Unit was safely transformed into a Nepali NGO and someone else was wrestling with the hospital issue. As already noted, my former student and friend Dr Arjun Karki had started a new Medical School under Kathmandu University. This was confusingly situated not in Kathmandu, but initially in Banepa and later in Dhulikhel to the east. At the time of opening the school, he invited me to join his teaching staff, but I was not free at the time. However in 2003 I accepted his invitation, just before going on home leave. As we were about to return, however, he emailed me to explain that he was likely to resign from his post over a very serious disagreement that had arisen between him and the University authorities.

Though I served under him for about three weeks, he did resign and I had a lot of sympathy with his reasons, which I will not recount here. He wanted me to continue to teach there, though he had every intention of opening another medical school and hoped I would join him there! He did, as I have recounted, found the Patan Academy of Health Sciences, but some years after I had retired. I did give some classes and lectures on visits.

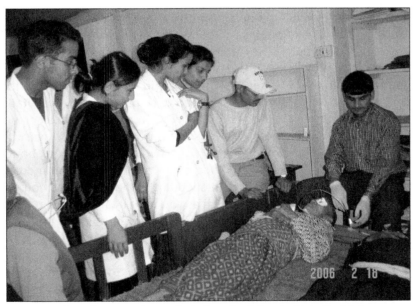

Medical Students, Kathmandu University School of Medical Sciences

Chapter 17.

Back to Nepal after 20 years with kids in tow. By Mary

Well, I'm really sorry. You thought you were done with me, with Mary Poppins rambling and all those forms of transport, but the old duffer (he'll edit that...) has asked me to do another chapter. Nepal revisited. If you were paying attention the first time you will remember I was just planning a trip with my husband and children. None of whom had ever been to Nepal before. I was a tad anxious, because to be honest I consider it a major character flaw if people don't like Nepal. The kids are picky eaters, and I wasn't sure how *daal bhat* would go down, but I was more worried about Andy. He said he'd be fine, as long as he could always get a cold beer. But in a country where load-shedding is the norm, and you're without electricity at least as much as you have it, and on a trip that included rafting and camping by a river, I thought this was a pretty steep requirement.

Fortunately they loved it. We had an amazing time, and it literally felt like the holiday of a lifetime. We were total tourists and we all loved it. Nepal had definitely changed in 20 years, however, so I got as many culture shocks as they did.

Kathmandu

Oh, it was good to be back. As I breathed in the totally unique stench of Nepal toilets in the admittedly perfectly clean ladies' loos at Tribhuwan airport, where 11-year old Abby had immediately repaired to vomit profusely, I knew I was home. (She has a thing with landing, if we make it out of the plane and to the loo, it's a major bonus... As we touched down in France one time, she threw up all over me, and in Denver all over the floor in the immigration queue.) As the stray dogs in the streets around the Kathmandu Guest House barked me to sleep that night, it felt like a familiar lullaby that I hadn't realised was missing.

As the taxi drove from the airport, though, I literally had no idea where I was. The city had expanded to the airport and beyond, and the roads were unrecognisable. As the taxi weaved its way past cows and temples, bicycles and people, I watched the kids' glazed expressions as they stared out of the windows. I couldn't work out if it was because it was all so different and unfamiliar, or if it was the effect of the long flight, the lack of sleep and the general vomiting. (Izzy had had a turn at the stopover in Qatar.)

They bounced right back though. When we emerged from our room on the second day, there was an Australian woman sitting wearily on the sofa on the balcony outside. "I'm so relieved I'm not the only one mad enough to bring teenagers to this country!" she exclaimed. "We've had tears." I was very proud of mine, who drank it all in, treated it as one long adventure, and assumed correctly they would enjoy it all.

As soon as we got there we set out for a recce around Thamel, the touristy part of town crammed with shops, money exchanges and hotels on chaotic narrow streets. I found it difficult to revert back from English caution, but the girls immediately picked up on how the locals do it, and darted across the roads in front of rickshaws and taxis, and weaved in between cows and beggars, relishing the chaos rather than finding it in any way intimidating. I'd forgotten the continual horn beeping, and the way your senses are assaulted by sounds and smells, pleasant and unpleasant in equal measure. Thamel itself hadn't changed all that much, and I was relieved that I could still find my way around, and the shops were every bit as enticing, to the girls' delight. We had our first meal in Nepal in the Kathmandu Guest House with the accompaniment of a Nepali band, and Andy tried his first Nepali *Thali*, (rice meal or *daal bhat*) along with a beer he allowed to be cold enough to be acceptable.

We were in Kathmandu at the start of the Seto Machendranath festival. I would say we were lucky to be there, but of course there are so many festivals in Nepal you would be pretty unlucky not to hit one of them. But we were lucky to see it at the very start. It's this huge tree-like structure built on a chariot and then pulled around the city, toppling precariously. There were men throwing gifts from the gods down from the top of this incredibly high construction. I was struck on the chin by an apple, which apparently was very auspicious, but frankly didn't feel like it at the time. It also rained as it set off, which apparently is also a very auspicious sign, but again, didn't really feel like a good omen for a holiday. The friend we were watching with said that, bizarrely, it pretty much always does rain. And it's not really the rainy season. The effect of the rain on the dust on the road led to mud splatters on my trousers from which they never recovered. Perhaps if it hadn't been 20 years, I'd have remembered white is NOT a colour for Kathmandu! I'd also forgotten the pressing crowds, the beggars tugging at various parts of your clothing and anatomy, the lines of people watching from the roofs, the lights strung around the temple area the chariot was first taken to, the extreme narrowness of the streets.

I thought my family were up to a minimal amount of sightseeing in the holiday of adventure that I had planned, and fortunately a kind friend spent a day chauffeuring us around in a tiny little car. We went up to Swayambhu, the temple on a hillock in the Kathmandu valley with a lovely view of the city and the hills around, and I was shocked to find another whole new shrine below it, with a towering glittering statue of Buddha flanked on each side by an equally towering Hindu god. The kids loved the monkeys, just as I had when I used to visit as a child. We went to Patan and admired the temples there, but I was disappointed that the temple square there is now a tourist attraction which you pay to visit, rather than being able to meander around at will. We had the happy notion of dealing with this by having lunch on a restaurant at the top of a 6 storey building from where we had an excellent view. Abby refused to try the *momos*, and went for the only thing she recognised on the menu; fish fingers. When they arrived she took one look at them and wisely declined to touch them. Andy ate them for her and spent an unpleasant night as a result. Retrospectively, ordering fish in a landlocked country with an intermittent electricity supply could be seen as an error! We had dinner that night with other friends, and by the end of the day I was overwhelmed and humbled as always by Nepali hospitality and generosity. That, it turns out, hasn't changed a jot.

Adventures to the West

The first of the adventures planned was rafting. We did a very similar trip to the one I'd done as a child (the "Never Know" trip if you have a better memory than I do) down the Trisuli river. Despite dire warnings from a friend who had been out more recently than I had, it really hadn't changed that much. I was expecting to have to weave down the river much like navigating the streets of Thamel, but we came across very few other rafts. The rapids seemed a bit tamer, but our guide compensated for that by playing a "game" that involved tipping us all out over and over again, and regularly letting us jump in to swim around the raft. (One of the kids' favourite memories is of me trying to get back in, and being hauled in by the back of my lifejacket like a beached whale.) The camping by the river was definitely more like 'glamping' than it was in the old days, but to be honest we were not complaining! It was a very beautiful camp, and if running water and electricity felt slightly like cheating, they were very convenient. And the (proper sit-down) loo had the biggest spider I remember ever seeing camped on its walls. We had a very happy couple of days paddling down the river to the cries of "Paddle high five!" and "Forward team!" from our guide, and were met at the take out point by our driver, Babu Raja, who was already becoming an old friend. I'd booked "private transfers" to and from rafting, and this turned out to be Babu Raja in a Land Rover who followed us round the country, turning up in unexpected places with a welcoming beam on his face, and hanging around for days at a time in more menial lodgings waiting for our next "transfer". One of my biggest fears about taking my family to Nepal was gratuitously ending their days over the edge of the Kathmandu-Pokhara road. Not without reason as it's a regular event, and indeed we saw one lorry on its side in the river as we floated down. However I never had any fears when we were in Babu Raja's hands. He'd actually wait until he could see the road ahead before overtaking, for example. Unheard of.

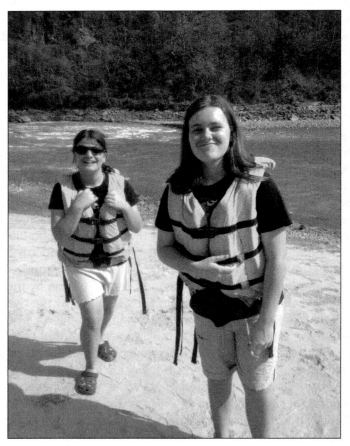

Rafting: Izzy and Abby

From rafting we went on to Chitwan, the flat jungle Terai land of Nepal. Slightly to my surprise this was the highlight. I knew the kids would like elephant riding, but I hadn't counted on the elephant bathing experience, and the most gorgeous lodge I've had the privilege to stay in. The Sapana Village Lodge lies by the side of the river,

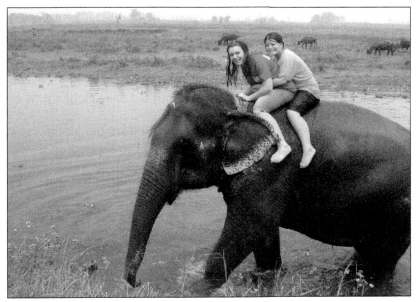

Elephant Fun and Games, 2014

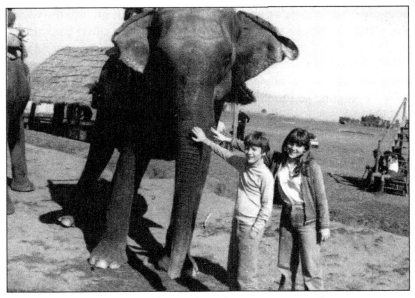

Compare Mother and Uncle many years earlier

with beautifully tended grounds with thatched houses for rooms. Hammocks lie strategically around the gardens, and terraces with bountiful cushions where you can lie sipping your drink, reading your book and watching the sun set over the river and the plain. It had the added advantage when we were there of not only having its own personal two elephants, but also a 3 month old baby elephant, with whom you could get up close and personal.

I had forgotten how excruciatingly uncomfortable an elephant ride can be! And, alas, the animals seem to have wised up to the tourist routines and we only saw a snoozing mummy rhino and her baby, a wild boar (also with its babe) and some deer. But the discomfort of this trip was soon forgotten in the joy of the elephant bathing experience. This is a whole new tourist wheeze that hadn't been invented when I was a child, and rivalled pretty much everything I've ever done in terms of sheer fun. Our lodge was out of the main drag, so our personal hotel elephant turned up to take just us to the river. No howdah this time, just the two kids and me bareback on this elephant, Abby and I clinging on for dear life to Izzy who was in front. The elephant walks down the bank (no idea how we stayed on!) and into the river. It takes a load of water into its trunk and sprays us all liberally. Then it kneels down and gently topples us off into the water. We scrub its leathery skin with a stone, and then climb back up its trunk by holding on to its great ears to start the process over again. (Well, when I say we climbed, the kids did it with no problem but once again Mummy failing to do so was totally hilarious!) Honestly I haven't laughed so much in years.

I should say it's not the most efficient way of getting clean and we all needed a shower afterwards!

Nothing could compare, but we followed it with a canoe ride and a "jungle walk" to admire crocs and birds and various plants, and a visit to the elephant breeding centre.

Spiders, geckos, mosquitos and hairy caterpillars all became mundane. We were very sad to move on from our jungle paradise.

Pokhara waited for us, however, and once again Babu Raja appeared on time, and with statutory Nepalese beam, to do the honours. Alas, Pokhara, once the most beautiful place on Earth, was hard to recognise. It used to be a rather small, deliciously hippy-ish town built by the shores of Phewa Tal (the same lake where I'd once left my skin behind in a kayak practising the Eskimo Roll.) The lake is obviously still there, but the town had grown beyond all recognition. I couldn't tell where I was, much to my distress, as we'd stayed in lodges by the lake so many times in years gone by. Most disappointing of all, the mountains hid from us almost the whole time we were there. I got up early every morning in case they made an appearance, and only once was rewarded. I woke Izzy; we had a strict rota for sharing rooms with Abby, who sleep walks/sleep talks/sleep argues/sleep shouts, making her an unpopular roomie, and it was just Izzy who blearily agreed to come down to the lake for an early morning boat ride. We hired a canoe to take us across Phewa Tal and finally I got to see my mountains, peeking over the shoulders of my 14 year old daughter as she paddled. By the time we returned and re-joined the rest of the family, however, they were almost all gone again.

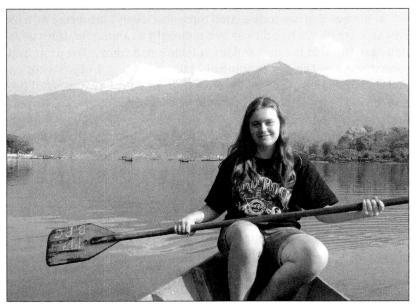

Izzy on Phewa Tal

I promised them all a gorgeous sunrise over majestic Himalayas looking close enough to touch if they agreed to spend one night in a lodge on Sarangkot, one of the hills above the Pokhara valley, but even then the mountains were hazy and unimpressive, to my intense disappointment.

However, there were compensations. The hotel we stayed in down in Pokhara was luxurious and boasted a swimming pool, as I'd thought we might need a bit of the kind of holiday they were all used to, but the lodge on the top of the mountain was much more in the style I'd been used to in my childhood. It was super-basic, perched right on the ridge, with the wind howling around it all night. The doors didn't shut properly and creaked in a sinister fashion, the taps dripped, dogs barked and mosquitos buzzed. Our beds were made up with traditional Tibetan lumpy duvet-type covers, and various insects and beasties joined us through the night. We were woken not only by alarm clocks telling us it was time for sunrise, but by the sound of hoicking and spitting from the owners performing their morning ablutions. It was perfect and I felt totally at home!

In the evening, we took a stroll through a lovely pine forest with its nostalgic smell. We had dinner by candlelight as a thunderstorm whistled past, blowing the prayer flags outside into a frenzy. The promised sunrise view, as I said, was somewhat disappointing, but we went up and down Sarangkot twice, because there are now two ways of getting down the mountain which made up for any lack of view. This confirmed Nepal as the coolest place (like) EVER in the girls' eyes. The first time we descended somewhat rapidly by the 'longest, highest, fastest zip wire in the world.' On the hour-long jeep trip up the first time, the couple we were with sang the praises of paragliding so effectively that we faced the jeep again in order to check it out.

I'd never paraglided before, and was expecting it to be pretty scary…like parachuting, where you appear to plummet for some time to your death before the parachute catches you. However, when paragliding, you get lifted off the side of the mountain into the currents, and you fly like a bird. Birds, huge birds of prey, were gliding right past your nose. It was, well, in the girls' words, epic. It was, once I'd got over the somewhat surreal feeling of having watched my 11 year old daughter throw herself off the hillside before me!

Nothing could compare to these experiences, but Pokhara offered us many more treats. Meeting my cousin (one of the Gerrards Cross ones if you were paying attention), who lived in Hong Kong at the time, and whom I hadn't seen for several years, but who by complete coincidence was bringing her own family trekking, as she had done herself as a child when they came out to visit us. Lots of shopping. Lunch at Boomerangs, a restaurant on the edge of the lake with a gorgeous view and delightfully mis-spelt menu. Discovering Moondance, our favourite restaurant, which nevertheless caused great distress to Abby when her cheese and tomato pizza came topped with (can you BELIEVE it?!)...tomatoes! Playing lots of games as a family. Following a herd of buffalo meandering down the main road (the girls found this hilarious, I was pleased to discover I hadn't really noticed it as unusual.) Being there for the start of Nepal's New Year 2071. (If you are reading this in the future, it was still 2014 for the rest of the world!) And, yes, a little bit of lying around by the swimming pool reading.

All too soon we had to catch the plane from Pokhara back to Kathmandu. Once again, I'd promised the family a beautiful flight along the Himalayan range, but all they saw was the cloud range. Back at Tribhuwan airport who should be there to meet us but the faithful Babu Raja. We returned to the Kathmandu Guest House for a final day. We spent this doing a bit more sightseeing and a lot more shopping. One of my school friends had got himself married to a Nepali rock star, and we spent the afternoon and evening with them and their son. We got to watch the band practice for a gig the following day, which was high delight for the kids, not sure Andy was so appreciative. [*Dad says:* This friend is the architect mentioned in Chapter 19 in connection with restoring buildings after the earthquake. We even saw him on TV in England!]

It was very sad to leave Nepal again, and it had all gone far too quickly, but I was so very happy to have shared it with my family. And even more happy that they had enjoyed it so much, and can't wait to go back. The highlights – watching our raft guide teach Izzy to write her name in Nepali in the sand by the fire at our river camp; seeing Abby in her "I love Nepal" t-shirt, adorned with Nepali merchandise; being soaked by an elephant; soaring like a bird over Pokhara lake; the competition between the girls for taking the best cow-in-the-middle-of-the-road picture; teaching them all Nepali phrases; introducing them to banana *lassi*; meeting old friends; the hospitality and the friendliness of the Nepali people. The frustrations – communication was the big one. In our world we are so used to instant contact with the click of a text or an email, but having to wait for electricity to get

Wi-Fi and the lack of predictability of texts arriving was hard to get used to. [*Mum says:* It used to take a month for a letter to get to UK if it didn't get lost on the way as many did.] And the mountains, of course, refusing to show off their splendour. There's nothing for it, I'll just have to take my family back again one winter. They won't say no!

Chapter 18.

Nepal; a potted history, 1969 to 2015

Before considering the ways in which the country has changed between 1969 and the present, I want to sketch in the political background to the momentous changes that we observed.

When we first arrived in 1969, King Mahendra was an absolute monarch, ruling through the partyless Panchayat System which he had established in 1962 after a brief attempt at multi-party government. He died in 1972 and was succeeded by his son Birendra. [*Angela says:* Many Nepali people wept profusely.]

A Constitutional Monarchy

The agitations around 1978-80 which so disrupted the training of the first batches of medical students, resulted in a constitutional referendum in which a small majority voted for the continuation of the Panchayat System and the King made some concessions allowing elections to the National Panchayat, though on a non-party basis.

However further campaigns, headed by the Nepal Congress Party and supported by leftist groups, increased in intensity until 1990, when, after major rioting, King Birendra agreed a new democratic constitution and elections took place the following year. He thus became a constitutional monarch, the first in Nepal's history.

The Maoist Insurrection

First the Nepal Congress Party and then the fairly moderate United Marxist Leninists were in power, but there was considerable instability. In 1995, the Communist Party of Nepal (Maoist) began an armed insurrection in the rural areas. For the next 10 years, the conflict between the Maoist rebels and the Royal Nepal Army formed the background to a succession of governments formed by different Prime Ministers. The rebels were responsible for ambushes, bombings, vandalism, *bandhs* (closure of roads, shops and businesses) and murders. They demanded 'political contributions' from travellers, including foreign tourists, and the tourist trade suffered.

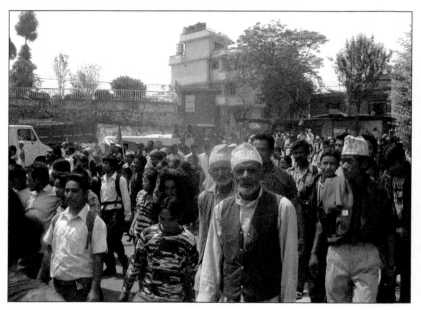

Maoist Rally

An extraordinary example of vandalism was as follows. The Maoists severely damaged a major hydroelectric generating plant, which had been built with Norwegian money and expertise, and put it out of action. Possibly because they realised they had lost public support over of this, the Maoists made an 'official' approach to the

Norwegian Government to pay for its repair! (I know about this because Jamie and I spent New Year's Eve in a trekking lodge on the Annapurna Base Camp route with, among others, the Norwegian Ambassador and family.)

The Maoist militia were strong in numbers, well trained and well concealed in mountainous and jungle areas. Military experts are well aware of the difficulties of fighting a guerrilla war against such an enemy, capable of blending in with a terrified local population.

The Royal Massacre

In April 2001, a general strike orchestrated by the Maoists, virtually brought the Kathmandu Valley to a standstill. However in June of 2001 came a dramatic and unexpected event which rocked the entire country, the Royal Massacre.

Conspiracy theories have been rife ever since, [*Angela says:* The Maoists promised an investigation into the truth. This has not yet happened.] The 'official' version propagated by the government is roughly as follows. The Crown Prince, Dipendra, was known to be unhappy with his parents because they were blocking his marriage to a certain Indian lady. On the evening of the 1st of June, having spoken at least once to the lady in India on his mobile phone and having taken a good deal of alcohol and certain unspecified drugs, he dressed himself in military combats, armed himself with a number of automatic weapons (which he kept in his rooms) and proceeded to an ante room where most of the senior members of the Royal Family were preparing to go in to dinner. He then opened fire upon them, killing King Birendra and Queen Aishwarya, his brother and several more of the assembled company. Having gone out into the garden, he shot at several more of his family and finally shot himself in the head.

Bizarrely, as he lay in a coma in hospital, he was proclaimed King the following day. However, he died on 4th June and his uncle, Gyanendra, took the throne.

Once he had shed the burden of absolute monarchy, King Birendra had become relatively popular. Not so his brother Gyanendra! Even less popular was Gyanendra's son and now Crown Prince, Paras. As Gyanendra had been one of very few royals absent from the palace on the night of the massacre and Prince Paras one of the few survivors,

177

it is understandable that conspiracy theories have considered that they were in some way responsible for the massacre.

Following the Royal Massacre, the Maoists again increased their campaign of violence. In November 2001, more than 100 people were killed in four days. Prime Ministers were appointed and fell. King Gyanendra took an increasingly active role in government, declaring a state of emergency and ordering the Army to crush the insurgents. This led to a great deal of killing but no weakening of the power of the Maoists. Peace talks were held and failed.

In February 2005, the King again declared a state of emergency and assumed executive power over the country. At first, people generally seemed to welcome this; the politicians had achieved nothing. However by November the main political parties and the Maoists were beginning to form an alliance with the main objective of overthrowing the King. They formulated this, of course, as 'restoring democracy'.

A Republic!

Following another round of peace talks, in November 2006, the Maoists and government signed a Comprehensive Peace Agreement. This marked the end of the insurgency, which had lasted 10 years, and in April 2007 the Maoists joined the government. Following an Act of Parliament, Nepal was formally declared a republic and the King became a private citizen. To the surprise of many, he did not leave the country to enjoy his riches abroad as had been expected, though his son Paras did move to Thailand.

As with the so-called Arab Spring countries, the removal of the 'tyrant' did not lead to an immediate state of peace and light. The political scene has continued to be turbulent, with dissent arising around several major issues.

One important issue was the fate of the members of the Maoist militia. Initially some 20,000 of them were kept in camps, supervised by UN personnel, but it was finally agreed that they should be integrated into the Nepal Army (no longer the Royal Nepal Army!) After the 10 years of bloody conflict, the Army itself was not keen on this as can be imagined. Eventually a belated and rather limited integration was decided upon.

A Secular State

At the same time in mid-2006 that the King's political powers were stripped from him, the government declared Nepal to be a secular state rather than a Hindu Kingdom. Part of the motivation for this was to divide the sense of nationhood from the monarchy and to weaken the tradition that the King was worshipped as a god. There may also have been international pressure about human rights and religious discrimination, but, since Nepal has always been particularly resentful of being told what to do by other nations, I suspect the internal reasons were the true ones. This probably marked the end of official persecution of Christians in Nepal, though it had been weakening in practice for some years.

Elections 19 November 2013

An important function of the elected multiparty government was to draw up the constitution of the new republic and the government became known as the Constituent Assembly. Between 2006 and 2013 governments rose and fell over the question of the nature of the proposed federal republic. The essence of the problem is the distrust that lies between the various ethnic groups in Nepal. These ethnic groups are not located in tidy geographic locations, but mixed throughout the country. It is true that certain tribes are found most commonly in certain areas, but the overlap is considerable. There has long been resentment, particularly among the Madeshis, people of the Terai, against the 'NBCs'; the Newars, Chhettris and Brahmins who had dominated the political parties for so long and who are also found widely scattered through the country, both in the hills and the Terai. The number of political parties increased enormously, many representing localised areas and their issues. So, while it has been generally agreed that Nepal should be a federal state of local governments, the actual method of dividing the country has been highly contentious. Some would like to see provinces divided without regard to ethnicity but many believe they will only get fair representation if governed by their own sort. But the extent of the geographical overlap appears to make this impossible!

An election took place on 19 November 2013 to elect the members of a new Constituent Assembly. Some seats were decided on a First Past the Post (FPTP) system and the remainder by Proportional Representation (PR). One hundred and twenty two parties took part in the election, with 10,709 candidates for 601 seats. Because of the level of illiteracy, ballot papers represented parties by symbols (animals, moon, stars etc.), so they consisted of 122 pictures.

Thirty three parties boycotted the election, led by a dissident Maoist group. They tried to disrupt the election, but apparently with limited success as a 70% turnout was reported. Some ballots had to be recast, however. The election was overseen by international observers, including former US President Jimmy Carter. They declared themselves satisfied with the conduct of the election, though the main Maoist party cried 'foul' after suffering a major defeat.

The Nepal Congress (NC) party won in both the FTTP and PR sections of the election, but by only a small majority over the Communist Party of Nepal (United Marxist Leninist). In spite of their name, the latter seem to behave more like a social democrat party. The United Communist Party of Nepal, (UCPN) the original Maoist party, came third in an ignominious defeat. *'Alu khayo'* as Nepalis would say; the party 'ate potatoes'!

Nearly two years later, in mid-2015, the Constitution had still not been proclaimed as there had not been agreement on the precise form of government and, especially, the number, names and divisions of the potential provinces. The mainstream Maoists and some of the Terai parties have been vigorous in their demands for ethnically-based provinces, while the Nepal Congress and the UML have been keen to avoid this. Dissenters had been demanding 'consensus', which for them means getting their own way in spite of being a minority in government. There were violent scenes in parliament as Nepal pursued its individual approach to democracy, including an undignified episode of chair-throwing.

The disastrous earthquakes of 25 April and 12 May 2015 might have been expected to put the constitution business on hold as the country entered emergency mode and then began the massive process of re-building homes, lives, infrastructure and food supply. There was considerable criticism of the government response as being late, inadequate and unduly bureaucratic in relation to foreign aid.

Possibly as a distraction from this, there was actually renewal of activity in moving towards a Constitution. Some politicians argued that a new Constitution was essential to enable the government to lead the re-building of the country.

Eventually, on 17 September 2015, Parliament voted by 507 votes to 25 to accept a constitution in which the country was to be divided into 6 provinces which would choose their names at a later date. This might sound like a final resolution, but dissenting parties, especially in the Terai, had boycotted the vote and continued to protest and disrupt national life. The President, Ram Baran Yadav, signed the Constitution into law on Sunday 20th September. In spite of protests from Hindu leaders and monarchists, the country is to remain 'secular'.

The Indian Government has protested about the constitutional proposals, which is understandably regarded as unwelcome interference in Nepal. The objections centre on the Terai and the Madeshi people who are related to Indians over the border and frequently intermarry with them. This raises citizenship issues for their spouses and offspring. Also the present Indian government is a Hindu Nationalist one and would like both India and Nepal to be Hindu states. In October 2015 the border with India was closed to supplies for Nepal. This was clearly disastrous with the homeless still not re-housed and winter coming on. It had not re-opened by the end of 2015.

Chapter 19.

Has it changed much?

Loss of Innocence?

The *Loktantra Andolan* or People's Rebellion of 2006 was a momentous turning point, though it was the result of a long process. In 1969 we found a Nepal generally at peace within itself and content to follow the hereditary monarchy which had been restored less than 20 years previously. People had a simple trust and a respect for authority, though most respect was given to leaders from the same ethnic group. It was close to being the poorest country in the world and most of the population consisted of subsistence farmers. They lived off their own land and made annual long journeys on foot carrying produce to sell if possible in Kathmandu or in India and carrying back essential supplies for their families. Of industry, there was virtually none. Most houses were of timber and mud or brick with a roof of thatch. Apart from one tortuous road to the Terai and India there were few hard-topped roads. The 'International Airport' was primitive and there were only a few grass airstrips in the rest of the country.

With only local radio and no television, there was very little understanding of the outside world. Cinema halls were few and only in cities. I recall a cartoon in the local newspaper when television first became available; the household TV was shown with a lighted candle on top of it! Very few people ever thought of going abroad, partly because it was so unknown and also because crossing the *'kalo pani'*, the black water, meant defilement to a Hindu. (The Gurkhas needed a special dispensation from the *pundit* in the early days of their service abroad.)

Two single lady missionaries were trekking though the hills and fell in to conversation with some local ladies. They were asked, as usual, how old they were, but had learned to handle the apparent rudeness of this question and recognised that it was standard politeness in Nepal. They were not prepared for the next question, "How many children do you have?" When they replied that they had none, the Nepali ladies looked amazed and one said to her friend "Don't they have children in their country?" to which the answer came "No–it's too cold!"

[*Jamie says:* One of my favourite culture clash moments was when I rode my friend out to Kalimati on Dad's Yamaha, with UK reserve about using the horn. Ivan asked me in all seriousness and without a trace of irony "I noticed that you don't use the horn much – are you a homosexual?"] Dad can't explain this.

I was lying under the stars with a porter on a trek in 1971 when we spotted a satellite making its steady way across the heavens. "Look–a star walking!" said the porter and I tried to explain that it was a man-made object that had been fired into space, but my companion would have none of it. Foolishly, I went on to tell him about the moon walk of 1969 and this he flatly refused to believe.

[*Angela says:* I like the story told by Georgia Rice. Her husband worked in agriculture in Okhaldunga. They set off to walk from Okhaldunga to Kathmandu, there being no road. Neil Armstrong got to the moon and back before they got to Kathmandu.]

In the schools, much of the learning was by rote and there was little equipment. Relatively few children attended, especially girls. Literacy was low, about 23% overall and only 2% among females.

There were few doctors and most of them were in the Kathmandu Valley. Infant and Child Mortality were high. Many women died in childbirth or with subsequent infections. Infantile tetanus was common, because of the practice of rubbing cow dung onto the umbilicus after the cord was cut. Though the disease was on the point of being eradicated, the scars of smallpox were to be seen on faces throughout the land.

Life expectancy was low; 42 years for men and less for women which is the reverse of the situation in most countries.

Road building

We have observed steadily increasing road building activity. Some are imposing highways, such as the East-West Highway which crosses the country in the Terai. The road from Kathmandu to Pokhara, though quite good, is a typical winding hill road liable to blockage by mudslides or the collapse of a complete hillside during the monsoon season. On one occasion, we were going for a family holiday camping and kayaking on Phewa Lake in Pokhara and had a kayak, paddles, tents and camping equipment all on the top of the bus when we met one of these severe landslips. There was nothing for it but for people in the long line of Pokhara buses to walk across the landslide, carrying all their possessions, and board a bus in the equally long line of buses facing in the opposite direction. Because of all our equipment and the difficulty of turning the buses in a narrow road, this made for a very long journey time.

In recent years there has been a tendency for smaller, un-surfaced roads to be gouged out of the hillsides to join villages to larger roads and towns. These are even more vulnerable to landslides. I was walking with a friend near Dhulikhel one day when we came across a team of workmen rebuilding one of these roads. We got chatting and said "Surely this will all come down again next monsoon?"

Back came the reply with a big grin, "Yes and we'll get paid to mend it again!"

With the improvement in the transport system, and perhaps largely because of it, has come urbanisation, a massive movement to the towns and cities. Kathmandu has spread out to the ring road, which used to run though rice fields and open country, to reach up to and beyond the foot of the surrounding mountains. Many former rice fields have been turned into smoking brick factories, surrounded by unsightly pits from which the clay has been dug. Increasing population has also contributed to the growth of the towns and cities; from just over 11 million in 1969, the population is now nearly 30 million.

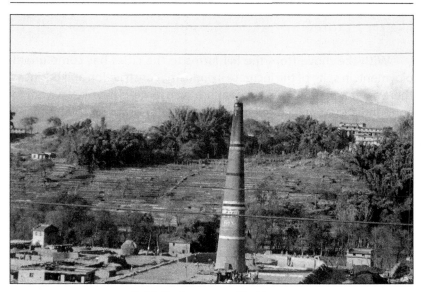

Brick Factory, near Bhaktapur

Historically, potential British Gurkha soldiers have been recruited from hill villages by former soldiers called *'gallawallas'* who march them to the recruiting centre for selection. They were youths who had been brought up working in the hill farms and carrying loads up and down hills day in and day out. Such boys were highly valued for their hardihood, strength and endurance and many were the sons, grandsons and nephews of former Gurkhas, so they had a sense of tradition and loyalty to the Brigade. Nowadays, however, the Gurkhas who retire build or buy themselves houses in towns such as Pokhara, Dharan and Damak, so their sons are brought up to a town life and no longer have the standard of fitness that the Brigade requires. As a result, the prized family tradition is getting weaker. On the other hand, with the improvement of education, the recruits have better English and mathematics and are easier to train for trades such as signals and clerking. There are now 'academies', run by ex-Gurkhas, that provide training for boys who want to try for selection for the Gurkhas.

Migrant Workers and the Diaspora

With the move from the hill farms to the cities has come unemployment. In spite of the increase in industry, construction and business, there are not enough jobs to go round. Even farmers have been wont to go to India for employment during the quieter times on the farm and have been prepared to do menial tasks, such as washing dishes in hotels and restaurants. They would be ashamed to be seen doing this work in Nepal. Still more striking has been the number going to the Middle East on a longer term basis to work in construction and other labouring jobs. The airport is thronged in the mornings with hopefuls waiting for the flights to Qatar and other Arab states in the Middle East. (We have benefitted from this, occasionally being upgraded to Business Class by the airline hoping to cram in more migrant workers in Economy!)

Sadly, these migrant workers are often cheated by employment agencies in Nepal or exploited by employers in the Middle East. Quite recently there has been a scandal in Qatar where large numbers are employed in construction work for the 2022 World Cup football stadiums. Some had not received pay for months, others had their passports confiscated to prevent them from returning home and some had been required to labour all day in the heat without being provided with drinking water. Following exposure of these abuses, the government of Qatar is said to be investigating.

Notwithstanding these abuses, many have found satisfactory employment and send part of their wages home to family in Nepal; the so-called remittance culture.

More qualified and educated people work hard to get the necessary papers to work in the USA, UK, Australia, China, South Korea and other developed countries. This results in a regrettable 'brain drain' and I am distressed when my former students or colleagues go abroad to do medical or nursing work. However some do return after further training and experience. Non-resident Nepalis (NRNs) have formed associations in a number of countries.

In Britain, we have ex Gurkhas and their families who now have a right to residence visas and also a quota of refugees of Nepali origin who were expelled from Bhutan and spent years in camps in Nepal. Putting together all these locations, there is an extensive Nepali Diaspora.

A More Demanding Society

Nepalis have learnt to protest! Though political protests had occurred earlier, the Maoist insurgency escalated protest from rallies, peaceful protest and civil disobedience to the overt use of violence. Not only the Maoists, but all political parties learnt the power of the '*bandh*' to try to get their own way on a wide variety of issues. The technique is to declare a *bandh* for a particular day or days and enforce it by means of gangs of thugs. These would be made up of paid 'rent-a-mobs' or members of the student union belonging to whichever party was protesting. If a shop opens on a bandh day, its windows are likely to be broken and perhaps its stock looted. If a vehicle of any sort is seen on a road, it may be attacked, damaged or burnt and the driver may be injured or even killed.

In 2002, there were 39 days of *bandhs*. I was quite surprised that the land of the Gurkhas so meekly accepted the restrictions imposed by the *bandh* but can see that it is a form of terrorism that puts fear into the hearts of the community. Still, as an observer and an expatriate, it seems to me that a concerted refusal to comply could put an end to this disruption for good and abolish a practice that is an obstacle to the prosperity and development of the nation. A Nepali economist recently estimated that each day of *bandh* costs the nation 3 billion rupees (about £190 million, US $300 million).

For a description of what it is like in a *bandh*, albeit a hastily imposed one in response to an external atrocity, please see Appendix III, 'Raging in Kathmandu'.

Others have also found that obstructing roads is a good method of getting one's own way or of obtaining funds. One example is found when there is a road accident in which local villagers are (or perhaps are not) injured. The villagers erect a road block and demand sums of money from travellers as a 'compensation' payment or for medical expenses. This is reminiscent of the Maoist 'political contributions'.

Schools

The development of private education has been a major feature of the change in Nepal that we have observed over the last 45 years. Ragged children used to walk up to 3 hours over the hills to a one- room bare school for their lessons, (providing they could be spared from work on the farm and parents realised the importance of education). Nowadays, the current pattern is more likely to be the school bus picking up groups of uniformed children in different parts of Kathmandu, snarling up the rush hour roads as it manoeuvres around dozens of other buses doing the same thing and delivering its human load to a private school. Here, many of the teachers are Indian and the fees high. In fact I am told that Nepalese with money to invest are most likely to invest it in private schools. Having said this, the standards of education are much higher than they were. One piece of evidence of this that we have observed for ourselves is the much-improved standard of English in entrants to nursing and medical schools.

In 1969 and for some years after that, Nepali was the only permitted medium for instruction. Nowadays, the private schools conduct their teaching mainly in English and even forbid the use of Nepali by the students. Incidentally, private schools are generally known as 'boarding schools', irrespective of whether they provide accommodation for the students, which mostly they do not.

In spite of this growth in the private sector, overall literacy rates are currently still of the order of 73% for males and 48% for females and in 2011 secondary school participation was only 46% for males and 38% for females.

Health

The government has considerably extended its system of Regional and District hospitals, Health Centres and Health Posts, but there is an on-going problem of providing qualified staff in the remote areas. Nepal now produces enough doctors for the needs of the population, but migration of medical personnel abroad and the concentration in towns and cities means that many of the Districts have far from sufficient medical staff.

As in the case of schools, the cities and towns have seen a huge rise in the development of private hospitals (generally called 'Nursing Homes', which conjures a different image for those of us from the UK). There are also private clinics without beds that may be manned by one or more doctors and situated in the premises of a 'Medical Hall' or pharmacy. The majority of doctors in private practice also have government appointments and have to find ways of juggling these two aspects of their lives. Needless to say, this generates accusations and conflicts, but it is true to say that many of the governmental and private facilities are delivering a very good service. The crucial point for patients remains the ability to pay, for even in government clinics, it is usually necessary to pay for medicines and supplies.

There have been some very good improvements in public health over the years, though much remains to be done. In 1969, best estimates were that between 25% and 50% of children died before the age of five years. This had declined to 139 per thousand in 1990 and 48 per thousand in 2011. Immunisation targets have been largely reached, between 80 and 97% in most cases. Life expectancy for men had risen from 42 years in 1970 to 65 years in 2012, by which time women's life expectancy had gone from below men's to 67 years.

Following the opening of the first medical school at Tribhuwan University in 1978, others have followed and there are now some 16 medical schools in the country. However some of these are primarily profit-making concerns that train a majority of Indian students who will return to practise in their own country.

Although nursing was considered a lowly profession when we first went to Nepal, it is now very popular and large numbers of girls apply for a much smaller number of places each year. (There are almost no male Nepali nurses.) Bachelor and Master Degree courses are also available. Like doctors, many seek to work abroad but they find it less easy to obtain places and visas.

[*Angela says:* Nurses often find work in care homes in the UK. Those who have remained in Nepal are Matrons or Campus Chiefs in nursing schools, and are making important decisions as members of the Nursing Council.]

Shopping, Business and communications

When we first went to Nepal, the only things available in shops were local produce and a few imported goods from India or China.

[Angela says: "You could often not even get sugar. The local alternative was a sort of sweet tasting rock crystal, '*misri*' that you had to bash into smaller pieces. (Sounds a bit like 'misery', which was appropriate!) It was a shock to have to make baked beans by soaking beans overnight and making your own tomato sauce. The flour had to be sieved to remove weevils. You had to toss the rice to get rid of the stones and chaff. You had to make your own butter from cream. Staying alive was hard work and time consuming. If you wanted toast and marmalade, ideally you would bake the bread, though an unpalatable loaf was available, make the butter and make the marmalade."]

Now the small local shops have been replaced by 'Supermarkets' in which foodstuffs, electronics and other manufactured goods are available from all over the world. Only beef is difficult to obtain, but not impossible, though it tends to be called 'fillet'.

When we first needed passport photos for trekking permits, we went and found a photographer in the street in Dilli Bazaar. He had an old camera on a tripod and disappeared under a sheet to take the photo. One arm would stick out; on a bright day, it would remove the lens cap to expose the film, wave it in the air once and then replace it. On a dull day, it would wave the lens cap twice! Today, needless to say, there are a lot of very advanced photographic studios with the latest digital technology.

For many years, the only way to make an international phone call was to wait for a long time to be connected from a public phone in the Central Post Office under the shadow of the Bhim Sen Tower. The arrival of ISD made a huge difference. Nowadays, most Nepalis in Kathmandu are seen clutching mobile phones. From our point of view in communicating with UK, the advent of email made a very big difference; no more waiting for 3-4 weeks for a reply to an airmail letter and not being sure whether or not it had got lost on the way.

The Earthquakes

How have the 2015 earthquakes changed things? We have not been in Nepal to observe it, but clearly there have been countless personal tragedies, with injuries, loss of life and the destruction of homes. UN figures indicate 8,617 people killed, 16,808 injured, 470,000 homes destroyed, 2.8 million people displaced and a total 5.6 million affected. More than a million have been in need of food assistance. There has been severe damage to the road system and communications and many villages have been completely cut off for long periods.

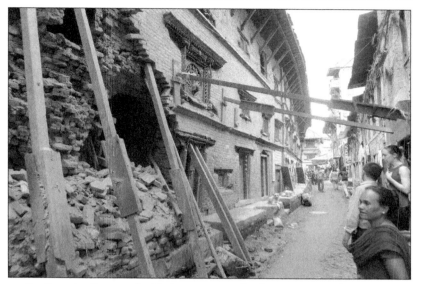

Earthquake Damage in Bhaktapur near the famous Peacock Window.
Photo: Jeanette Happ

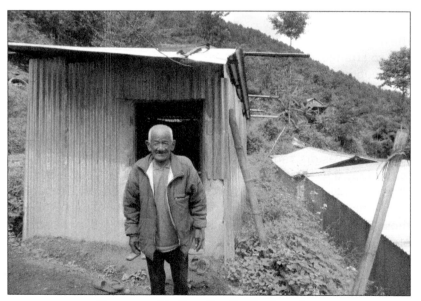

Temporary Shelter after the Earthquakes.
Photo: Jeanette Happ

Though less important for national life, there was much publicity about the many mountaineers who were stranded high on Mount Everest as a result of avalanches that swept away the route through the notorious Khumbu Icefall. Mountaineering, trekking and tourism are only gradually recovering and the long term effects are uncertain.

Historic buildings, many still showing the effects of damage from the 1934 earthquake, have been destroyed or extensively damaged (including the Bhim Sen Tower, or Dharahara, near the old central post office where we used to try to make phone calls to the UK). One of Mary's school mates is now an architect with major responsibility for the restoration of these buildings; it will be a lifetime's work. We hear that Shanta Bhawan, the old hospital and home for many of our Nepali friends, has been destroyed.

We are thankful that none of our closest friends was killed or severely injured. With one exception, their homes are more or less intact.

Finally

I was on one of my assignments in Nepal for the Army and had the amazing experience of attending a Christian Easter Day parade. Not so strange, you may think, but this was the first year that any such public expression of faith had been allowed. There were thousands of Christians in church groups, carrying banners, singing hymns and rejoicing in the living Jesus. I hope my many Hindu friends will forgive my feelings about this; we had gone to Nepal in 1969, a time when there were only 500 Christians country-wide, many of them foreigners. Pastors and new Christians were frequently imprisoned. In the crowded New Road, I had so many times felt that I was perhaps the only Christian in all that throng. Now there are probably a million or more Christians country wide. I was deeply moved to see those great crowds freely worshipping their risen Lord in the streets of Kathmandu.

We missionaries (old-fashioned word though that may be) took no credit for this miracle; it was the Holy Spirit, working through a handful of Nepali believers, who brought about this change. Nepali Christians are peaceful and co-operative and they want nothing but good for their homeland.

But these Christians have discovered something special that they want to share. They, too, want to 'serve the people of Nepal in the name and spirit of Jesus Christ'.

Appendix I.

Twelve New Doctors for Nepal (1984)

This appendix is taken from an article I wrote in the British Medical Journal
(Dickinson, J, 1984)Br Med J (Clin Res Ed) 1984; 289 doi: http://dx.doi.org/10.1136/bmj.289.6460.1715 (Published 22 December 1984)

What is a doctor, anyway?

W hat does a general practitioner have in common with a forensic pathologist, or a neurosurgeon with a clinical biochemist? Increasingly little in these days of specialisation, yet their basic medical training and qualifications are likely to be similar.

Almost as different as the spheres of various specialists are the spheres of work of doctors in developed and developing countries. Arriving in Nepal in proud possession of my membership in 1969, I found that I had to relearn my profession in a most painful way in order to be the sort of doctor that Nepal needs. Not merely different diseases, but different priorities, different social structure, and different attitudes to health and disease make medicine in Nepal a specialty of its own. As most Nepalese doctors are trained in neighbouring India, you might expect them to find it easier to cross the cultural and professional gap between training and service. Not at all. In fact, coming from medical colleges run on similar lines to the most traditional of British schools, these doctors find medicine in Nepal even more of a shock than I did, especially when, as usual, they are posted initially to a remote area. A Nepali doctor writing on this says, "They were never trained for such an alarming situation. Their role model was entirely different." So he was–the consultant head of a hospital team using advanced technology. Clearly the challenge facing the planners was to define a Nepali doctor in terms of the competencies required of him and to proceed to train doctors in Nepal to fulfil this job description. I hope to show that the curriculum that emerged from this process is no less demanding than a traditional one; it simply has different emphases and priorities.

Overcoming the demands of those who urged a traditional medical school, the Institute of Medicine of Tribhuwan University in Kathmandu took the first steps to meet this challenge in 1977 and prepared a plan for an innovative medical education programme. By August 1978 the plan was complete and the first batch of students was admitted to the course, then named rather clumsily the "Diploma course for the degree of doctor of community and general medicine," but now renamed, by decision of Tribhuwan University, the "MB BS course."

Defining the product.

The aim of the programme is to prepare community physicians who will serve in the health services for at least four years as medical officers in the rural areas with three major roles.

- A clinical role to save life, to restore health, and rehabilitate by providing medical care in a district hospital.
- A preventive role in maternal and child health, environmental health, nutrition, health education, communicable disease control, and school health.
- An administrative role, collecting and updating appropriate demographic and epidemiological data, planning and implementing comprehensive health care in the district, functioning as leader, and ensuring the effective functioning of the health care team in the district.

The reader may care to pause and ask himself how he would like to take on this job description and how the breadth of these requirements compares with the depth of knowledge required in his own particular discipline. To help him do so, let me paint a rough picture of the position in rural Nepal. It is a mountainous land in which travel by foot is the rule; almost any route means at least three hours' continuous steep ascent; socioeconomic development is low; infant mortality is among the world's highest, around 140 per thousand live births; the under 5 mortality is between 25% and 50%; the population growth rate is 2-6%, and Nepal has the lowest arable land to population ratio in the developing world. The disease pattern is just what you would expect in a land that lacks safe water supplies, sanitation, and hygiene, and where rough terrain, population pressure, and traditional practices combine to prevent adequate nutrition.

Philosophy of the course

So far eligibility for the course has been confined to those who have had at least three years' experience in delivering health care in Nepal. They have had about two and a half years of training at the Institute of Medicine and then served as health assistants, pharmacists, radiographers, laboratory technicians, nurses, or Ayurvedic (traditional) practitioners according to their training.

This requirement has ensured that candidates are familiar with the health needs of Nepal and allows the selectors to judge how they have withstood the pressures of these needs. In contrast to the technical emphasis of most medical courses, there is a strong emphasis on community health, which occupies the students' attention for the first six months and then continues as a thread throughout the course. This underlines for the student the object of the training—the health of Nepali people, not the manipulation of calcium channels or the control of the rejection of transplanted tissues. It was intended that the course should be "integrated" in various ways; curative medicine with preventive care, basic medical science with clinical medicine, and the four sciences of anatomy, physiology, pathology, and pharmacology with one another to give an integrated approach to the systems of the body.

So far as possible, a self-learning and problem based approach has been adopted. In the systems study, for instance, students are given clinical problems and are required to analyse them on the basis of their knowledge of the basic science involved and their own experience. Community problems, such as population control are tackled in the same way. As we have seen, doctors cannot be defined on the basis of a common body of knowledge or skills, but they do have in common the ability to solve medical problems. It seems only right that this should be a major thrust in medical education. Classes are kept small; only 22 students in the first two batches, increasing to 30 in the third and fourth batches. Students of other courses are working on the same campus and the students are encouraged to view doctors as members of the wider health team. The course is divided into three phases over a period of four years followed by a year of hospital internship

Problems and difficulties

Administrative difficulties and the lack of a fixed university calendar led to the loss of about a year for the first batch of students who lost an additional 18 months of study time as a result of student agitation in which they were caught up, for the most part, unwillingly. They therefore took their final examinations after six and a half years. Poor facilities put a strain on faculty and students. Classrooms were primitive, water and electricity supplies irregular, visual aids few and difficult to use, and the library inadequately stocked and limited in reading space. For clinical work, the students were sent to busy hospitals where heavy service commitments made it hard for doctors to give them adequate attention. Many of these problems are likely to disappear with the opening of the Tribhuwan University Teaching Hospital, the excellent classrooms of which are already in use and which is expected to admit its first inpatients in October 1984.

At the outset, there were important gaps in the faculty, especially in the basic medical sciences. As these were filled with difficulty, one by one, the teachers developed curriculums for anatomy, physiology, pathology, and pharmacology independently of one another and integration suffered accordingly. We all of us suffered from inexperience; we had received our own training in very different courses

198

and, although ideas had been borrowed from various recent experiments in medical education, none of us had any experience in implementing them.

Subjective view and the physiology course

All the above problems were eclipsed by the sheer enthusiasm and motivation of the students and the freshness of this approach to medical education. Small classes are also attractive, though a class of 22 presents great difficulties when it comes to dividing it into small groups. I deliberately concentrated on clinical aspects of physiology and biochemistry, using mainly measurements that are feasible in a district hospital. No oscilloscopes, no nerve muscle preparations, no complex biochemical analyses. The students' bodies provided the experimental material and I used patients to argue from disordered to normal body function. I wanted the students to have a good working knowledge of body function and control mechanisms and not to become bogged down in conflicting theories of detailed mechanisms. There was consequently little emphasis on the history of physiological discovery and experimental method. The students were encouraged to read up these aspects if they wished; it would be relatively easy for them to gain experimental ability at a later stage if necessary. I like to think that my own sense of wonder at the complexity and sensitivity of bodily mechanisms communicated itself to the students. In April 1984 the results of the final examination for the first batch of students were announced. Of 22 students admitted to the course, 21 took the examination having passed all previous exams at the first or subsequent attempt. Of these, 12 were successful and the remainder will repeat the examination later. I was present as an observer at the clinical and oral examinations in medicine of some of the students. The standard of history taking, physical examination, and diagnosis was extremely high. X-ray examinations were interpreted well and there was no difficulty in describing the use of various implements. Questions were in English and the answers were generally accurate in content, though the use of the language was often clumsy. External examiners, two from India and two from Canada, were impressed. One Indian asked to take some of the graduates back to his hospital in India and was politely but firmly refused. A

Canadian said that the candidates compared favourably with their counterparts in his country.

As the successful 12 begin their internships, I and my colleagues at the hospital already think that they are better prepared for the work than graduates of Indian medical colleges who have completed their internship programmes. Needless to say, they should be much superior in rural and community work. The future

If initial enthusiasm has, as I believe, overcome the extreme practical and logistic difficulties, the prospects are bright. It will be important to maintain the vision, to resist the pull to conform, to shun inappropriate technology, and to train new, young teachers into the programme. Facilities are improving, experience has been gained, and the "product," the first batch of graduates, exists as a creditable example.

The possibility of postgraduate studies has been discussed from the beginning. If the present standard is maintained or improved, there is no reason why teaching centres abroad should not be persuaded to accept Nepalese graduates after a short period of reorientation.

Students often ask me, "Will we be as good as doctors in the West?" This takes me back to my original question: what is a doctor? Moreover, what is a good doctor? The graduate of a London teaching hospital is doubtless superior in ordering and analysing a wide range of tests, but how would he manage a rural hospital in Nepal? I have no hesitation in telling my students that, for Nepal, they will become not only as good as Western doctors, but immensely better.

Appendix II.

Death and Dying in Nepal (1983)

This appendix is taken from an article I wrote in the British Medical Journal
(Dickinson, Death and Dying in Nepal, 1983)Br Med J (Clin Res Ed) 1983; 286 doi: http://dx.doi.org/10.1136/bmj.286.6363.471 (Published 5 February 1983)

The delicate relation between a doctor and the relatives of his deceased patient seems to differ from country to country and from age to age. Apparently in ancient China it was the custom to execute the doctor if the patient died, a practice that doubtless promoted either careful medicine or meticulous selection of patients. In Britain, so far as I can recall, a comfortable attitude of mutual understanding prevailed; the doctor would offer some attempt at consolation and the relative would respond with, "Thank you, doctor, I know you did your best." In the USA the response is more likely to be, "You may have done your best, but I aim to sue you anyway," an attitude that must bring out the defensive and suppress the compassionate in the doctor.

Here in Nepal medical litigation is mercifully unknown, but we experience faint echoes of ancient China. There is a definite element of resentment against the doctor for his failure, though the Nepalese are too polite to put this into words. Regular attenders at the clinic default suddenly after a death in the family and, in some hospitals at least, the wards may empty like magic after a death. The message is plain: "Results count. Dead patient means bad treatment."

Understanding the 'Ghat'

If the doctor cannot save the patient, the least he can be expected to do is to ensure that the patient is discharged in time so that he may be taken to a "*ghat,*" a sacred cremation site by a river, before the death occurs. This could not be more different from the Western custom. Imagine the psychological effect on a patient of taking him to the graveyard before he dies. Relatives here, as elsewhere, are unwilling to tell the patient directly that he is dying, but will make the same statement at the last moment by taking him to the *ghat,* if necessary against the doctor's advice. I have no objection to referring to the *ghat* the old, the incurably ill, and the undoubtedly dying, but I find a serious moral dilemma with the young patients with potentially curable infectious disease for whose survival I would like to struggle to the end.

Whose patient?

But whose is the ultimate responsibility for the patient anyway? As a physician I like to feel that in time of illness the responsibility is mine; that is what I have been trained for. Not so in Nepal. It still seems strange to me when a relative comes to me and asks, "How is my patient, doctor?" I feel like replying, "He is your relative but my patient," but it is better to keep quiet and learn the Nepalese attitude about such things. In their view, the patient remains firmly part of the family and they do not expect any emotional participation on the part of the doctor. If the patient dies, why should the doctor feel grief? Why should he offer consolation? The patient belongs entirely to the family and their minds are now full of their grief and of the arrangements for the cremation that must be performed at once amid all the rites prescribed by the Hindu Vedas and the traditions of the caste. Any failure in the performance of these rites carries the same inauspicious meaning as a death occurring in the hospital rather than at the *ghat*; both lead to difficulty in the passage of the departed soul to the next incarnation. In the belief of some at least, this could rebound on the family in the form of a malevolent spirit that would bring bad luck on the family and only be exorcised by extensive further rites.

Consoling the 'inscrutable'?

Contrary to the image of fatalistic inscrutability projected by romantic writers about the East, I find Nepali people far from dispassionate about death. Indeed, there is much less attempt to conceal grief than you find in Britain and the wailing of the women can be heard all over the hospital in spite of the attempts by the nurses to prevent or dampen it.

Here then are many reasons why I find it virtually impossible to offer any consolation; I am held responsible for both the death and its inauspicious location; I am shut out from the family; I cannot penetrate the wailing grief. Even the option of a sympathetic hand on a shoulder is closed to me as such physical contact is culturally unacceptable.

In an active medical unit treating advanced disease in a developing country, three or four deaths in a day is not uncommon, so it is clearly important to come to terms with this problem, but I am not sure that I have yet done so. As I turn away from the bedside and leave the family to handle their grief, I feel guilty that I cannot be of any help to them, that I can find no culturally acceptable way of supporting and consoling them. Probably my main trouble lies in trying to apply the cultural expectations of one society to another and I would be better simply to accept things as they are.

Occasionally, I get it right. The retired military gentleman was my oldest patient at 93, which is more than double the life expectancy in Nepal. Despite a variety of disabilities his enjoyment of life was undiminished, though he showed a certain forgetfulness, such as addressing me in Hindi rather than Nepali on occasion. When I was summoned to the house and found him suffering from a respiratory infection, I was prepared to transfer him to the hospital and try to save him. A brief family conference, however, decided that the old man's time had come. My experience had by then shown that Nepalis are often uncannily right in such things, so I agreed to his being taken to the river where he died within a few hours. With their usual graciousness, the family credit me with having predicted the time of death with miraculous accuracy. As for me, I do not recall having attempted any such prediction. They miss the old man. So do I and our relations remain intact.

Is all this leading to any conclusions?

Yes-leading to conclusions that we should all have reached in our medical schools, but somehow they got obscured in the rush to ascertain the necropsy findings and we have had to learn them by experience since. Even the best of doctors loses patients, and the more active the unit the more frequent are the deaths. Death is a family matter and we need to be sensitive to the personal, social, and cultural needs of the family. These needs may be different from those of our own society. (This must be an important aspect of practice in Britain now as there are increasing numbers of Muslim, Hindu, and even Buddhist families.) When a doctor cannot prevent death, he can and should ensure that the conditions surrounding the death are compatible with the dignity of the patient and the cultural require-ments of the family. In almost any society, death in hospital is less likely to provide these conditions than death at home or in the cul-turally appointed place.

Should not we hospital doctors pay more attention to these things instead of regarding death as a failure and a threat?

Appendix III.

Raging in Kathmandu 2004

This appendix is adapted from an unpublished essay that I wrote in 2004, when I was motor cycling daily to the Kathmandu University Medical School, then situated in Banepa, nearly an hour's ride to the east.

September 1st.

T oday started inauspiciously. It was dark and wet and I had to make an 0720 start on the motorbike to reach Kathmandu University Medical School in time to give an 0830 class. I had read on the BBC website the night before an unconfirmed report that 12 Nepali hostages, migrant workers in Iraq, had been executed by the extreme Moslem group that had captured them. However I had not anticipated the strength of the Nepalese reaction or the degree to which Nepal has taken to violence and destruction as a response to any perceived insult.

After my class a student asked if I had seen the video of the beheading and shooting of the hostages; it was being shown more or less continuously in the Library. I had not, and I did not. Shortly after, another student asked if I was about to go home. I was not. Then came increasing reports of violence in Kathmandu; strikes, road blocks, burning tyres. One of the buses had arrived to take staff to Kathmandu, the other never came. Most of these staff members were preparing to stay overnight locally in Banepa or Dhulikhel. Then came news that a curfew had been announced in Kathmandu, so no-one could return there anyway. Additionally came an announcement that the government had declared the following day a public holiday. As it happened, Angela soon phoned me to confirm that things were tense in Kathmandu and her Nursing Campus had closed, but that the curfew was to begin at 1400 and I had better set out straight away if I was to get home before it was imposed.

So I set off for the 17 mile ride home. It was 'interesting'. The first event was a demonstration going on in Banepa, near to KUMS. It looked like a political demonstration, with waving of flags and shouting slogans, and it was more or less surrounded by police. The roads beyond that were noticeably empty; very few buses, some motor bikes, but fewer than usual.

Approaching Bhaktapur, I came across the first barrier of burning tyres across the road and they became more frequent as I approached Kathmandu. Some were blazing merrily, but most were smoking and dying down. There were a couple of halfhearted attempts to stop me, but I pressed on. Though there was little traffic, there were large numbers of people walking or standing around.

In a couple of places, the police gestured me to stop. I showed my white face, gave them a cheerful "good afternoon" in English and continued–they are not usually interested in stopping expatriates, especially if they think they will have to speak English!

Approaching home, on the ring road, I came across the worst signs. Bigger burning tyre barriers and some more substantial blockades, though all proved negotiable. Then a dead body. I do not know the story, I just saw a middle aged woman, poorly dressed, lying in the road with some police and a small crowd looking on. Then there was some rock-throwing. I don't think it was at me, but at two cars that were overtaking me.

Then onto narrower roads, almost deserted, and home. I waited to hear if other prevalent rumours were correct; aggressive crowds at the few Masjids in Kathmandu, a Moslem cleric killed, three deaths at a place called Koteshwor that I pass each day.

September 4th.

Things are now a bit clearer, though the last 3 days have been highly confused and we have mostly been confined indoors (as has our houseguest!). The curfew is still in force, though lifted a few hours a day to enable people to do some shopping. The death of an imam has not been confirmed, though there was a good deal of damage and fire at several mosques. Nothing about the deaths at Koteshwor, though one protestor was killed and others injured. This will doubtless be ascribed to police brutality and will cause future protests. The death of the lady on the ring road has not been mentioned. Manpower company offices (deemed to have improperly sent workers to the Middle East) were attacked and looted. Few seem to have escaped, whether or not they deal with the Middle East. Inexplicably, newspaper and TV offices were also attacked and the security forces took little action. There were attacks on Middle East airline offices and flights have been suspended.

Why?

National pride, certainly, but there seems little doubt that certain political parties took the opportunity to discomfort the government through their student branches. The government was accused of taking insufficient action to prevent the executions. Also, many young Nepalese have aspirations about going abroad and earning big money and their hopes took a major blow. None-the-less, the extent of this reflex recourse to violence and civil disturbance is bad news for the future of the country. As the churches insist, the hope of the nation is in God alone.

Isaiah 17:12   New International Version
Woe to the many nations that rage— they rage like the raging sea!
Woe to the peoples who roar— they roar like the roaring of great waters!

Appendix IV.

Running the Ring Road (1981)

This appendix is taken from an article I wrote in the British Medical Journal
(Dickinson, Running the Ring Road, 1981)Br Med J (Clin Res Ed) 1981; 283 doi: http://dx.doi.org/10.1136/bmj.283.6300.1180 (Published 31 October 1981)

The Ring Road

For a capital city, Kathmandu is quite small. Chinese aid, however, has provided it with a ring road–broad, well-built, and almost entirely free of vehicular traffic. Perhaps one day, when the city has sprawled beyond it, the ring road will serve the purpose for which it was intended. Meanwhile, its broad grass verge will continue to attract those of us who like to run.

[*Update:* My forecast proved correct! The Ring Road is almost unrecognisable now, surrounded by buildings and choked by lorries, buses and every other sort of traffic. To run on it now might prove fatal!]

Reaching the ring road can be a problem as I stumble over the rough, stony path, trying to avoid people and animals. The children, particularly, stop to gawp at the now familiar sight of the British doctor pounding the paths. They have a small vocabulary of shouted comments. *"Kuire"* apparently means nothing more obnoxious than "paleface," but when they use *"bandar"*, which means "monkey," they are liable to get their ears cuffed.

Jogging or Running?

The ring road is empty by comparison but there are some pedestrians, including old ladies carrying huge loads of cattle feed (I have nightmares about being overtaken by one of them).Today, I will just run a small segment and return by another path but on two occasions companions and I have run a full circuit of the city, a distance of 17 miles or 27 kilometres. Our last time, two hours and 25 minutes, seemed very respectable but I was discouraged a few days later when Nepal's top distance runner covered the full marathon distance of over 26 miles in a slightly shorter time. In common with others, I object to the verb "jog" in this context. Surely it is a transitive verb; my elbow or my memory may be jogged but the ring road certainly shows no sign of being "jogged" by me. What I do is to run. I really do not know if running is going to preserve the patency of my coronary arteries or keep my weight down or my blood pressure normal. I do it because I like it and feel better for it and because it helps me to feel like a young man. In the hot sticky days before and during the monsoon, I wonder if I am being a bit masochistic, but in the winter, under the blue sky and with the glorious Himalayan peaks peering down on me, there is no doubt that it is pure pleasure.

Reflections on Physiology

Nepal is in the process of producing its own medical graduates for the first time, and one of my challenges is conducting the physiology classes for the students. I cannot claim to be a physiologist, just a clinician "with an interest .. ." as the advertisements say, but I have always been awed by the adaptations that the human body can make to different activities, conditions, and demands. If I am not too exhausted I like to reflect, as I run, on the changes my body has to make between leaving my outpatient desk and running along the ring road.

What has really caused my ventilation to increase? Is it the input from my tortured joints that has stimulated my respiratory centre? Or has there been a minuscule rise in my arterial PCO_2 that has stimulated my central chemoreceptors? Or might I just have a small remnant of innate, non-reflex common sense that has caused me to breathe harder? At what point on my longer runs do I change over from metabolising carbohydrate to breaking down my fat stores? Should I succumb to the temptation to wipe my face with the bottom of my vest or would it help my heat loss mechanisms if I were to leave the sweat to evaporate? What, I often wonder, is the reason for the increased lower abdominal cramps and urge to defecate that I, and others, often suffer during running? Surely the parasympathetic system is well damped down during exercise? Being a mild asthmatic with a moderate exercise-induced component, I have yet another physiological matter to ponder. Sitting at my desk, it is relatively easy to visualise those beta receptors at the bronchial smooth muscle cell surface, their stimulation to increased adenyl cyclase activity, the intracellular increase of cyclic AMP, the activation of a protein kinase, and the resultant muscle relaxation; running the ring road, the action of my salbutamol inhaler seems pure magic.

Though I have not managed to convince my students, increasing numbers of city Nepalis run. Village folk, on the other hand, are faintly amused at the phenomenon. They, of course, get more than sufficient exercise digging their fields, carrying huge loads up and down the hillsides, and covering great distances to fetch supplies or to visit shrines on the tops of distant hills. Because of their high energy output and relatively low food intake, fat villagers are almost unknown. I am interested in their attitude to fluid intake: however long the journey, however steep the path or heavy the load, they rarely drink water. By comparison, my mouth feels like sandpaper under such conditions and I top myself up at every stream or spring. They tell me that it "makes you sweat" to drink on the trail, which I suppose has some physiological truth, but is not the relative dehydration too high a price to pay? Is this the reason that they often complain of dysuria, constipation, and dizziness? Running with others is a delight, and this way I often learn new routes. Usually I set off with my son or with colleagues from the hospital, but sometimes a solo run becomes companionable as a local Nepali joins me. We all have our different strengths and weaknesses in terms of stamina, speed, uphill running, and tolerance of wind and heat, but it is usually possible to modify the run so that we are more or less together at the start and finish, and everyone gets the exercise that he wants.

Memories

Memories of old runs come back to me as I near the end of my ring road segment. Port Meadow in Oxford was pleasant and relaxing but I will never forget the heavy sand of a West African beach as I tried to get fit for university rugby football at the end of a student elective. Perhaps my biggest disaster was the run I took at Banff in the Canadian Rockies at 6 am before a day of medical meetings. Clearly I underestimated the Canadian winter, for in 20 minutes I managed to freeze my fingers and ears. When the time came for me to present my paper, I had great difficulty in managing the slide changer, the electric arrow pointer, and the podium light. This was an embarrassment since the topic of the symposium was mountain medicine.

Now I am off the ring road and approaching the final hill before home. The path is crowded, my bowel is cramping, and my airways' resistance is increasing again. A final sprint? Ah, well, perhaps this time I'll just settle for walking the rest of the way home.

Appendix V.

HIV in the Mountains (2001)

This is an article I wrote in June 2001 about the current state of HIV/ AIDS in Nepal. It was submitted for a special edition of the British Medical Journal but was not selected for publication. I have updated it with some recent figures at the end.

Until the middle of the 20th century, Nepal was isolated from the rest of the world. This was partly a matter of policy, but there were also physical barriers: the immense Himalayan range to the North and dense jungle and wetlands, with their accompanying mosquitoes and malaria, to the South. Now the jungles are gone and the southern border with India is wide open, to the extent that up to 1.3 million Nepalese men, driven by poverty, go out of the country each year to seek work. According to USAID, 94% of these migrant labourers from one district go to India and 33% of these to Mumbai (Bombay) with its heaving red light areas and high prevalence of HIV infection in the commercial sex workers (CSWs). In addition to this, there are believed to be some 200 000 Nepalese girls employed in sex work in India and other countries, whether willingly or having been "trafficked" against their will.

Origins and patterns of HIV in Nepal

We do not know how HIV entered Nepal originally. Was it through a tourist? Was it a returned CSW or migrant labourer? Was it connected with intravenous drug abuse? It seems certain, though, that all these routes are involved in the continuing spread of the virus. Nepal, of course, has its own sex industry and some, but not all, of the CSWs are returnees from India. The industry is generally not brothel-based, as elsewhere, but freelance. Girls operate in Kathmandu and other towns and in teashops and small hotels along major transport routes. This pattern is good news in that client numbers are relatively small, but the scattered nature makes it difficult to target interventions.

Nepal also has its intravenous drug users (IDUs), possibly 30 000 of them. They are concentrated in the cities and towns and the prevalence of HIV among them is 40-50%. There is interaction with CSWs. Though homosexuality is a taboo subject, there is no clear evidence that it is a major factor on Nepal's HIV scene.

Though supporting figures are not available, it may be useful to think in terms of two epidemics, one urban and based on indigenous commercial sex and intravenous drug use and the other mainly rural and fed by the sex industry in India and elsewhere through labour migration.

Numbers

Reported figures are minimal; around 2000 cumulated HIV positives and 500 AIDS cases since the first report in 1988. However the estimated actual number of HIV positives in Nepal is about 34 000. WHO/UNAIDS classifies the epidemic here as "concentrated", that is with prevalence more than 5% in population sub groups (CSWs and IDUs), but low in the general population as measured by prevalence in ante-natal clinics.

The big epidemiological question is "Will the epidemic become generalised in the way that it has in African countries?" By definition, Asian countries such as Thailand and Cambodia have generalised epidemics (HIV prevalence in urban ante-natal clinics >1%), but the prevalence of HIV in the general population (2% and 4%) is much lower

213

than found in Africa and is thought to be declining. It is possible that this is explained by the fact that the epidemic is younger in these countries than in Africa, and by effective interventions. However, it is more likely that the reason is to be found in lower sexual exchange ratios in the general population in Asian than in African countries.

So what can we expect in Nepal?

The best predictions are for 1-2% prevalence of HIV in the age group 15-49 years by 2010, unless effective interventions can be implemented. This would not be as devastating as the situation in many sub-Saharan African countries today, but would mean something like 10 000 to 15 000 AIDS patients, a burden far beyond the coping ability of the health infrastructure.

What is being done?

There is a National Centre and District AIDS Committees. There are many non-government organisations (NGOs) doing good work, most dramatically in rescuing girls from the sex industry, sometimes even snatching them as they are taken over the border. Some provide services for IDUs, treat STIs, and are active in awareness raising and counselling. The problem is that they are all in limited areas and have limited capacity. They (we) do the right things, but without sufficient reach, even in Kathmandu.

My own Unit has worked in awareness raising in the 1100 workers and their families in the various projects of our mission organisation. As many of the projects work in community health, non-formal education and rural development, it has been possible through them to disseminate the message about HIV prevention quite widely. A rough survey showed that in 3-4 years, the most successful of the projects trained in early batches had reached the following approximate numbers of people.

Furthermore, of 55 staff members who had received training, 52 said that they had talked to family and friends about HIV and AIDS and the total number spoken to was an astounding 4615, or an average of 89 per staff member.

Project	Number reached
A Rural Health Project (W)	18 000
An Urban Health Project	11 000
A Rural Health Project (E)	5 000
A Hospital in a hill town	10 000
A Hydropower Project	8 500

In addition to this, we work in counselling training and also help in the development of care and support of AIDS patients in health facilities.

Like everyone else, we have not reached enough people. Those we have reached are probably not in the highest risk groups, though we may have reached some potential migrant labourers. However, our Training of Trainers system, cascading knowledge out to the community, appears promising at least from the quantitative point of view.

Nepal is not alone in needing more government commitment, a stronger health infrastructure and more resources to combat HIV. There is a highly successful DOTS programme for TB, which could provide a matrix for an HIV network, and there are some tottering steps towards co-operation.

I have not mentioned anti-retroviral treatment as it barely exists. If it did, it would suck resources from other urgent needs, as basic as clean drinking water. It should come eventually, but I hope it will be in a planned manner, so as to be effective, properly resourced and monitored to avoid the propagation of drug resistance. We should implement a DOTS-like programme from the beginning, and not have to fall back on it when random therapy has failed. There are similarities between HIV and TB treatment, but two big differences: HIV treatment is not finished within a few months and it does not, in itself, contribute to controlling the epidemic.

Finally, we need a major intervention programme aimed at harm reduction among the sub populations at highest risk, IDUs, CSWs and their clients. Such a programme is beginning, albeit more slowly than we would like. As well as promoting condom use, needle exchange and the treatment of STIs, it will have to come to grips with the way that HIV crosses that long, open border. India is no more "to blame" than any other country or people for the wildfire spread of HIV, but it is clear that, without concerted action on both sides of the border, the fire cannot be extinguished in landlocked Nepal.

Update 2014

Though still representing a great deal of human suffering, the actual course of the epidemic has been less severe than predicted in 2001. Estimated prevalence in 2014 for the age group 15-49 was only 0.2% rather than the 1-2% predicted and it appears to be falling. The estimated number of people living with HIV in 2014 was 39,000, though only a third of these are diagnosed. 10,407 people were on Anti-Retroviral Treatment (ART).

References and Bibliography

Probyn, M. (2011). *The Living Goddess.* Kindle Books.

Dickinson, J. (1981). Running the Ring Road. *British Medical Journal*, 283.

Dickinson, J. (1983). Death and Dying in Nepal. *British Medical Journal* , 286.

Dickinson, J. (1984). Twelve New Doctors for Nepal. *British Medical Journal*, 289.

Heath D, Williams D, Dickinson J. (1984). The Pulmonary Arteries of the Yak. *Cardiovascular Research*, 133–139.

Lindell, J. (1979). *Nepal and the Gospel of God.* United Mission to Nepal.

Paton, A. (1981). Mission to Belsen 1945. *British Medical Journal, 283*, 1656-8. doi:doi.org/10.1136/bmj.283.6307.1656

West, J. B. (1982). *The American Medical Research Expedition to Nepal 1981.* The Himalayan Journal. Retrieved from http://www.himalayanclub.org/journal/american-medical-research-expedition-to-everest-1981/

WHO. (1987). *Hospitals and Health for All.* WHO. Retrieved from http://apps.who.int/medicinedocs/documents/s17390en/s17390en.pdf

Steele, Peter. (1972). Doctor on Everest. Hodder & Stoughton

Would you like to help Nepal?

There are many ways of helping. Some organisations find good ways of meeting needs described in this book. They can be found as follows:

United Mission to Nepal Hospitals Endowment Trust.
Pays for hospital treatment for poor patients in Patan, Tansen, Okhaldhunga and Amp Pipal
www.umnhet.co.uk. See Chapter 4.

Toilet Twinning. (Tearfund)
Helps overcome the lack of hygiene that leads to diarrhoea, typhoid, hepatitis and other water borne diseases; this is an amusing way of helping build toilets. www.toilettwinning.org. See Chapters 2 and 6.

United Mission to Nepal.
Active in many ways, based in Kathmandu
www.umn.org.np

International Nepal Fellowship .
Active in many ways, based in Pokhara
www.inf.org.

Gurkha Welfare Trust.
Financial and medical aid for ex- Gurkha soldiers and their families in need
www.gwt.org.uk. See Chapter 15.

Index

CPSIA information can be obtained at www.ICGtesting.com
Printed in the USA
BVOW11s0954220216

437604BV00005B/5/P

9 781498 461221